THE POWER WITHIN

True Stories of Exceptional Cancer Patients
Who Fought Back with Hope

WENDY WILLIAMS

A Fireside Book
Published by Simon & Schuster
New York   London   Toronto   Sydney   Tokyo   Singapore

Fireside
Simon & Schuster Building
Rockefeller Center
1230 Avenue of the Americas
New York, New York 10020

First Fireside Edition 1991
Published by arrangement with HarperCollins
Publishers
10 East 53rd Street
New York, New York 10022

Manufactured in the United States of America

10 9 8 7 6 5 4 3 2 1 Pbk.

Library of Congress Cataloging in Publication Data
Williams, Wendy.
    The power within: true stories of exceptional cancer
patients who fought back with hope/Wendy Williams.—
1st Fireside ed.
        p.   cm.
    Reprint. Originally published: New York:
Harper & Row, © 1990.
    "A Fireside book."
    1. Cancer—Psychological aspects. 2. Cancer—
Alternative treatment—Case studies. 3. Mind and
body. 4. Mental healing. I. Title.
RC262.W554   1991
616.99′4′0019—dc20   90-28138
                                                        CIP

ISBN 0-671-73790-2

Contents

For Mary Jane,
    who said this book would happen,
        and
For John,
    who made it happen.

Preface

This book is about finding courage. It tells the stories of ten
people with cancer who were terrified but who gradually replaced some of that terror with a new knowledge of life and of
spirit. Slowly and often hesitantly, they confronted their fear and
found special, unexpected resources within. Julie calls those
resources "love." Lisa calls them "hope." Smadar, once an
atheist, calls them "God."

One man, Bob, calls these unexpected resources "the
perverse benefits of cancer." No one, Bob says, would willingly
choose to have cancer. But if cancer is given to you, there are
important gifts that can come to you as well.

Every person in this book initially felt overwhelmed
and victimized by the diagnosis of cancer. But each gradually
learned that there is life after cancer, and that there are still
opportunities for choice and change. "Choice" is the key
word here. The choices may be major—which cancer
treatment to undertake or whether to continue work—or the
choices may be subtle—how to deal with a friend who has
not called since the diagnosis or what kinds of foods to eat.
But the choices are there, giving you the ability to take back
control of your life.

Each person in this book believes he or she has free choice. "Choice" does not mean the choice of whether to have or to give up cancer. "Choice" means how a person decides to live after the cancer diagnosis. Lisa, faced with that decision, initially chose to pull the hospital bedcovers up over her head, hoping the doctors at her bedside would just disappear. Later, in a cancer support group, Lisa met two important people: a woman who had become embittered and reclusive because of her illness and a man whose love blossomed as his lung cancer grew. Lisa learned she had a choice about how she would live with cancer.

The people in this book are sometimes fearful, sometimes angry, sometimes filled with grief. But they are never passive. Not one of these ten people once used the phrase "cancer victim" during our conversations. They do not think of themselves as victims, either in their cancer experiences or in the rest of their lives.

These stories are all true. They are not meant as formulas for action—if you do this, this, and this, then that will happen. These are not stories about people who adopted a macrobiotic diet and got cured, or about people who meditated and got cured, or about people who found God and got cured. These stories will not tell you how to cure cancer.

These stories are meant to show the wide range of possibilities that exists in our lives, and they address the issue of healing rather than curing. These stories tell us that anything can happen, that miracles do occur.

But miracles are not always obvious. A miracle may be the complete and unexpected recovery of a woman hovering on the edge of death. Or a miracle may be a gift of love and faith left by a young wife to sustain her husband. The miracle may also be less dramatic but of great consequence: A workaholic father strengthens his relationship with a distant daughter after diagnosis of a brain tumor, or a woman with two lung lesions spends her days gathering and delivering food to be distributed by Mother Theresa's nuns in San Francisco.

What do these miracles mean? That there is more—much more—to life than the surface view. In each of these stories, cancer has helped people look under the surface, into the deepest layers of existence.

And what they found there was hope. Hope is defined differently by each of these ten people, and will be defined differently yet again by you and by me. Is it possible, then, to say that any of these definitions are wrong, invalid, or false? After talking with these ten people, I believe there is no such thing as false hope. After hearing these stories, I believe calling another person's hope false is a tremendously arrogant action.

When I had nearly finished collecting these stories, an acquaintance at a party asked what the book I was writing was about.

"Cancer," I answered.

Her party face gave way to a stricken look.

"My mother's just been given six months to live. Well, actually the doctor gave her six months. But then he changed his mind and gave her a year and told her if she had any trips in her future, she'd better take them now. So she and my dad are off in Hawaii."

I told her about Bob, alive and jogging two years after being told he had four months to live; about Ray, who at 60 was at the peak of physical condition after four major cancer surgeries and who started to lift weights because a doctor told him he couldn't; about Lisa, who walked 10 miles to raise money for a hunger project after living with ovarian cancer for nine years; and about Sylvia, who held her first grandchild in her arms eight years after hospital medical staff urged her husband to make funeral arrangements.

This book is for the woman I met at the party, for her mother and father, and—most definitely—for that soothsayer doctor. Doctors cannot give patients months or years to live. They can only quote statistics.

Life is not controlled by statistics; statistics are only numbers. Life is a pact made between an individual being and the spiritual forces of the universe.

Only God can know the future.

Acknowledgments

This book belongs to all those who helped bring it into existence.

Most especially, the book is a creation of those ten remarkable beings who willingly discussed their most painful and most triumphant moments in life.

Nevertheless, there would be no book were it not for the unquestioning loyalty of Tony and Priscilla Parker.

Professionals from cancer support organizations throughout the country contributed time, information, advice, and, of course, support. Thanks to the Cancer Help Program of Bolinas, California; Norman Cousins of the UCLA School of Medicine; Cancer Coping Skills of the Ontario Cancer Institute of Toronto; Exceptional Cancer Patients of New Haven, Connecticut; Albey Reiner of the University of Massachusetts at Amherst; the Wellness Community of Santa Monica, California; and the Wellspring Center for Life Enhancement of Watertown, Massachusetts.

The people whose stories make up this book have used their real names. The events and places they describe are real, as are the names of their doctors. The names of a few other individuals have been changed to protect their privacy.

Ray Berte

INTRODUCTION

After Ray Berte had a total laryngectomy in 1973, his doctors warned him not to lift weights.

"You can't," a solicitous surgeon said. "When you raise them over your head, your shoulder blades will come together and pinch closed your air passage. You won't be able to breathe."

Ray had been a lifelong sports maniac. He played football in high school, played baseball with all the boys in his large family, loved swimming in the ocean. But he had never lifted weights. So, after hearing the warning, Ray ran over to the local gym and signed up for weightlifting.

Fifteen years and four cancers later—including one terminal diagnosis a decade ago—the handsome, black-haired Berte looks like a well-conditioned, muscular 45-year-old.

Actually, he's 60.

Ray's Story

One of the toughest lessons I have had to learn in my life is when to surrender and when to stand and fight. A macho American man, a real man, never gives up. If you do, you're a quitter.

Once, when I was a teenager at camp, two fellow counselors decided to throw me into the pool.

"No way," I yelled at them. "You two guys are never going to get me into that pool."

We were good friends, but soon we were rolling around on the ground, absorbed totally in battle for its own sake. The boys came at me and I wrapped my arms around a large tree with thick, rough bark. I kicked with all the power of the adrenaline and testosterone raging inside my adolescent body. They pulled, tugging me around the tree. My fingernails ripped; my face bled; I cried and cried inside, although those boys never saw the tears.

They never got me into that pool. After a half-hour they gave in. They finally quit; I was victorious. But I was a bloody mess.

Now, with the maturity that comes of facing my own death, I wonder about that day long ago. Wouldn't it have been better, wiser, to have given in and ended up with clothes that were wet instead of bloodstained and ruined?

How many times in life do we do that kind of thing? We become addicted to fighting like that, so that fighting becomes more important than winning the war.

Cancer has taught me to step back and assess my battles. And now I allow myself the pleasure of surrendering, of giving up a battle, in order to win the much larger war of surviving on this earth and living a worthwhile life.

Don't misunderstand. I certainly don't mean giving up on the important things. When the doctors pronounced my bone marrow cancer fourth stage and gave me at the most two more years, I just wouldn't go along with them. I was ready to marshal my forces. I was 15 again with my bloody arms wrapped around that tree.

It took many years and several times under the surgeon's knife for me to learn what I'm trying to tell you. I'll start with this: I had one hell of a singing voice. Even today, 15 years after they cut the larynx out of my throat, I still grieve the loss of my singing. I listen to the tapes of my performances and I just can't believe my ability to sing was cut out of my life with the throat cancer. But it was.

Singing wasn't my whole life. I had a wife and two children (still do), and an associate professorship at Springfield College in the Rehabilitation Services Department (still do). But singing was what I *did*. The central focus of my life was to perfect my high C, to emulate the tenor beauty of a Franco Corelli.

In the spring of 1973, I was lecturing to students at the Hartford School of Social Work and suddenly I could barely talk. My voice became so hoarse that I just managed to finish the lecture. The problem persisted for several weeks and I could not sing, even for my own entertainment.

I visited an ear-nose-and-throat specialist.

"Well," the specialist said with relief after examining me, "at least it isn't cancer. It's some kind of virus that's settled on your vocal cords."

I was pretty annoyed with the guy for even bringing up the subject of cancer.

"These guys are all alarmists," I told my wife, June. "You know, knife-happy. It's nothing serious. I feel fine, except for the raw throat."

After several weeks I went back to the specialist, who called in his partner for consultation. They decided I should see yet another specialist. That specialist ordered a biopsy performed. The results were negative, but they sent me to Boston, to see yet another specialist at Massachusetts General Hospital.

He ordered a biopsy performed, with negative results. He ordered more tests.

My wife and I drove the two hours to Massachusetts General a second time in June 1973. As we walked into the examination room, the doctor's nurse turned her back on us.

"The doctor will see you now," she said, trying to get out of the room without looking at us. But I saw the tears.

Our Boston specialist said the words: "Malignant throat cancer. I've agonized over how best to treat you: a partial or a total laryngectomy. I've checked with several of my colleagues, and we think the treatment of choice is a total laryngectomy. It's not too bad. There are only two things you can't do after: sing and swim."

"You stupid fucking sonofabitch," my brain screamed. "What do you mean I can't sing anymore?"

That response was mental. Aloud, I said nothing. It was my first surgical procedure, the first time I heard the words "treatment of choice," and I just assumed the doctor's word was law: He prescribed, I obeyed.

Most people who get throat cancer get it because they smoke or drink too much alcohol. Or they smoke and drink alcohol at the same time—that's even more dangerous. Obviously, as a dedicated singer, I never smoked. And I rarely, rarely drank. So my throat cancer was strange and unusual indeed, one for the books.

No physician or scientist has a good medical theory about why I developed such an atypical case. I do. I remember my father constantly telling me that I made too much noise, pantomiming strangling me if I didn't quiet down when ordered. So, years later at age 43, my throat quieted down. I believe there are no coincidences in life.

A laryngectomy means the complete removal of the larynx, the voice box. You can't talk and you become a neck breather. There is a hole in your throat. Your whole life turns upside down.

The power of speech deserts you. I woke up from surgery,

July 10, 1973, in a large room filled with machines. There were women in white and patients screaming for attention. Plastic surrounded me; needles sat in my veins; pressure bandages grabbed my throat. I couldn't breathe, and I couldn't call for help. That organ, that function of my body, no longer existed. I tried to call out but the capability was absolutely not there.

"Come and help me," my brain bellowed. The words stayed silent.

Later on, I remember June standing with me, helping me. And I remember a strange woman, a speech therapist, yelling at me about getting out of bed and getting on with my life.

I went home from the hospital on July 24, full of terror that my wife would find me repulsive and that my children would not want to be around me. No one had told me that mechanical devices, electroesophageal devices, existed to help me get through the coming difficult period. I lived in a world of silence, communicating to my wife by writing messages or tapping in code.

The telephone rang. It was a day in August 1973. The phone rang and rang and no one was home but me. The insistent ringing demanded acknowledgment. I picked up the receiver.

"Daddy, Daddy, I'm sick," my eight-year-old daughter, Jennifer, was crying. "Daddy, please, please come and get me. Daddy, I want to come home. Please."

"I hear you, sweetheart," I answered. "You'll be OK. Mom and Dad will come to you as fast as we can and ease the hurt."

But she never heard me. The words stayed silent. My little girl called for my help and I couldn't answer.

I grabbed the keys to the car, trying to keep functional, and drove to where June was working. June called Jennifer, and together we went to pick her up. In the end, Jennifer came home and got over her flu, but I never got over not being able to respond to her hurt.

I absolutely knew I could not remain handicapped like

that. But learning esophageal speech had been presented in an incredibly negative light. When I was in the hospital, a doctor had asked what I intended to do for work for the rest of my life.

"Why?" I wrote on my magic pad. "I'm a teacher. I like teaching. I'll always be a teacher."

"Obviously," the man said, "you can't go back to teaching. If you're lucky enough to learn esophageal speech, it will take you two years, and even after that you can't talk more than 10 to 15 minutes at a time. It's too exhausting."

The message was clear from the medical world: No matter how hard I worked, I would never be able to regain a normal communication capability.

That was his diagnosis of my state. My diagnosis of his state: an acute case of the glass-half-empty syndrome. A lot of these medical types are infected with it. They train themselves to be tentative and negative and call it scientific. But since when does science say you have to believe in the worst? And why doesn't a man as intelligent as a doctor understand the incredible hypnotic effect of words, the lunacy of using "if"? You don't have to lie, just tell the whole truth: Some people use esophageal speech quite well. Even if the statistics are poor, you can still stress the positive.

I was also put off at first by listening to the esophageal speech used by several others who had had laryngectomies. They sounded so terrible, almost incomprehensible.

"If that's what I'm going to sound like," I thought to myself, "I'll stick to my pad and pen."

But I was saved by my stubbornness. I intended to speak to my daughter again. Myself, without any mechanical devices. Esophageal speech is basically skilled burping. You swallow air. You trap the air in your throat. You burp it back up, creating the vowels and consonants with that air. It's kind of like creating a whistle from the neck of a balloon; as the air escapes, you change the pitch.

I had to change my expectations from sounding like

Franco Corelli to sounding like a cartoon character. Instead of reaching the zenith of hitting a perfect tenor's high C, I had to settle for trying to sound the syllable "baa."

Every night after dinner I sat alone in my library, trying to say "baa." Then I struggled to get out my first word. When it finally came, I hadn't had the best of days. The word I said was "shit."

Every night in my library I sat at my desk and tried to read aloud the titles of the books on the shelves. Hour after hour I spent perfecting, eliminating extraneous noises. The process felt familiar even if the sounds were strange: For a voice student, sitting alone for hours vocalizing is part of a normal day.

Despite the medical profession, there were people to encourage me. Back at college, lecturing at first with an electroesophageal device, I was terribly self-conscious about being effective. I must have asked frequently if the students could understand me that first time, because suddenly the lecture turned into a revival meeting.

"You sound good to me, Doc," called someone.

"I hear you loud and clear, Ray," said another.

I didn't need to ask for encouragement after that; the students kept it up on their own. At the end of the lecture they gave me a standing ovation. I gained more from their hour of encouragement than I ever gained from all the doctors who have ever said "never" and "can't" to me over the past 15 years.

There probably aren't 12 people in the whole country who use esophageal speech as well as I do. And I learned it in three months. And I have lectured for an eight-hour day using esophageal speech.

My point is not to brag. My point is to tell you this: Only people limit people. That guy in the hospital didn't know. He only thought he knew. He didn't know me, and he couldn't see into the future. So how could he predict what would happen?

Push the limits when the battle is worth winning. If only one person in the world has achieved a certain goal, make yourself be the second. Or, if no one has ever done it before, let yourself be the first.

Gradually, June and I and the kids settled back into a routine of work, school and family life again. I missed singing, but thought I was adjusting. And the cadence of my esophageal speech was nearly identical to voiced language.

Then, a year and a half later in Florida, June felt a lump between my shoulder blades as she rubbed suntan lotion on my back. I tried to be protective of June and the kids, telling them it was nothing. But inside, I knew.

We went back to Boston, and the experts said they wanted to leave it alone to reevaluate it in three months. But on the way home I started thinking. Three months. I was not going to let that thing sit in my body for three months, growing and festering. I called my local surgeon and suggested a lumpectomy.

"Cut that damn thing out and let's get it under the scope," I said. The good news was that the tumor was another primary, without evidence of metastases. So now there's a big hole between my shoulders where the tumor used to be.

Then again, another year later, I noticed a lump on the side of my neck while I was shaving. Once again my local surgeon cut out the tumor sites, three lymphatic glands.

"They look innocent enough," he said, holding the glands for me to see in the outpatient clinic.

"Wanna bet?" I said.

The next day, I called for the results of the biopsy.

"We don't have them," the nurse said.

I called again the next day.

"We still don't have them," she said.

Cancer patients become so sensitive. I knew that sometimes those results are available before the patient is off the table.

"You have an appointment with the doctor Monday," was all the nurse said. "You be sure to keep that appointment."

Then I knew. Another cancer. This time it was lymphoma.

The stuff was running through my lymphatic system. But as cancers go, it wasn't so bad. Then the local oncologist suggested a bone marrow biopsy, as a precaution, I guess.

So I went in for an appointment with the specialist. My white blood count was skyrocketing, the guy said. "Not so good," the guy kept muttering, talking numbers and statistics but not really talking to me.

And then it came: "Fourth-stage bone marrow cancer." He tried to slip it in, and kept talking about numbers and stats. I called for time out, but he apparently hadn't heard me.

"Time out, dammit!" I said.

He stopped. But then he continued, using that phrase—"treatment of choice."

"Don't tell me about treatment of choice," I said. "Narrow it down. Say this is the best medical option. I can take that. But tell me what the options are. Tell me the pros and cons. I will make the choice."

This was the beginning of a new attitude toward what was happening. I stopped taking orders and started making decisions. I stopped thinking of my doctors as gods who would deliver me from hell and started thinking of them as merely one aspect of my own, self-designed treatment plan.

This gets touchy here, because some people will read this and think I'm telling them I have the answers, that if they do what I did, they'll live a decade longer than the statistics predict. Let me be clear: I'm not telling you that. There are no absolute answers. There is no magic bullet. There are no guarantees.

You have to do it yourself. That's the whole point of what I learned. The doctors can tell you, "This is what we think. This is what we suggest." But they don't know for sure. They only have statistics that produce mathematical suggestions. In the end, it's up to you.

That time—the third diagnosis of a primary cancer—their suggestion was experimental chemotherapy coupled with radiation. There were quite a lot of exotic, experimental therapies around, because nobody knew quite what to do with fourth-stage people.

I'm not against traditional medicine. After all, up to that point it had kept me alive. But this cancer was pretty much of a mystery to the medical world. And I didn't think I wanted to live a miserable, debilitated existence on the basis of medical betting.

So I decided to go it alone on this one. I decided to look into adjunct or ancillary therapies, the therapies outside traditional Western medicine. I said no to the radiation, no to the chemotherapy. I became very aggressive in seeking out knowledge. I read, visited clinics, talked to people nonstop. I was thinking there had to be some less invasive way.

The doctors didn't like it. The chemotherapy was absolutely necessary, they said, if I wanted to survive.

"This guy's chasing rainbows," wrote one cancer expert from Boston.

"If you take the chemotherapy, I will give you maybe two more years," another said.

That was when I realized we were playing by completely different rules. They were talking about giving me two years. I was talking about winning the war and becoming cancer-free.

Who wants to rely on a teammate who thinks you've already lost? The accusation that I was a rainbow-chaser was equivalent to saying, "Go drift into your never-never land. Die there, because that's what's going to happen."

"I don't know anyone ever winning a fight who felt he was going to lose before entering the fight," my high school football coach used to say.

I remembered him, and I remembered the guy who told me I couldn't teach anymore and the guy who told me I couldn't lift weights.

For my new teammates, I chose all the people before me who had survived fearful illnesses. I chose all the writers who had written about the human spirit. I chose organized, healthy exercise; a special, high-nutrition diet; family members who said they loved me; friends who believed I would be around forever.

"If you opt for the chemo, we'll probably give you a couple of years." The medical community kept up the pressure.

Immediately after that "couple-of-years" conversation, deeply depressed, I visited a close friend.

"Six to eighteen months?" he said. "Great! That gives us plenty of time to work this thing out."

I took the Boston expert who accused me of being a rainbow-chaser out of the game and replaced him with this friend.

I also took two weeks to go to a clinic specializing in adjunct cancer care, based outside the United States. At the clinic I learned a great deal about how to take care of myself, about meditation, about nutrition, about relaxing and about restructuring my stress-filled life-style. The doctors at the clinic were far from quacks; my primary care doctor had been a physician at a major Philadelphia hospital for 13 years, but had become tired of being hamstrung by the American medical world.

I'm not going to tell you the name of the clinic, because that's not important. It was not the clinic itself that turned me around. It was my belief in the clinic. And each person has to find that belief himself or herself. I can't say, "Eat macrobiotic food," or "Go to this clinic," or "Take that drug." You have to make your own decisions.

At the clinic, I found other believing patients, and our enthusiasm for each other helped carry us through. An older woman rode on the airplane with me from the United States to the clinic.

"Ray," she said, "young man, you're going to beat this. I know it."

I added her to my team.

So, gradually, I put together what I consider a full deck of cards in my favor. I have a sense of humor, a healthy life-style, and good teammates.

People call me "Miracle Man." I'm not. I'm just an average guy who got tired of thinking of himself as a "cancer victim." The third time around, after a pretty extraordinary set of circumstances, I said, "Enough. I'll do it myself this time." I took an aggressive posture, went out and gathered information, and made some decisions. I decided to take responsibility for my life and to use my recurring cancer as an opportunity for growth.

I don't know if the change in my attitude contributed to the length of my life. Maybe I would have died. Maybe not. There's no way to know.

But I know the change has contributed to the quality of my life. And I know I have achieved victory over cancer. I have become an initiator in life, instead of a responder. In Chinese, "crisis" carries two connotations: danger and opportunity. I decided to take advantage of the opportunity provided by the cancer. I've become a better father, better husband, better teacher. I risk more, cope more. My sensitivity to other people has increased.

You are not to blame for your cancer. But you can take responsibility for your life by saying, "What's my contribution to this situation and what can I do to change it?"

One of the best members of my team, by the way, is my oncologist, who has been with me throughout most of my cancer experience. When I started designing my own program, he took a risk and stuck with me. He let me know right from the start of the cancer that I could continue to live fully and vitally. He never predicted my death or told me what I couldn't achieve.

"I don't agree with what you're doing," he said when I decided to go to the holistic clinic. "But if you feel the need to do it, go ahead and do it."

He's been a big member of my team throughout everything. Ten years after the Boston doc warned me I would die,

I still have a high white-blood-cell count. It's lower than when it was first diagnosed, but higher than the average person's. So I visit my oncologist regularly, to keep up the tests and to monitor any changes. When I go, my doctor closes the door and we sit and chat about things at length. We talk about cancer and statistics; I tell him my disturbing and radical notions about health. We talk about sports teams and life and about people who have died recently. I think I'm a very bright spot for him, someone who beat the statistics with a little bit of help from my friends.

EPILOGUE

Ray experienced yet another cancer in 1987. Surgeons removed a testicle with unmetastasized cancer. Following that, Ray self-published To Speak Again, *a book about his experience.*

Ray's oncologist, Frederick Flatow, faculty member of Tufts Medical School and attending physician at the Bay State Medical Center, said Ray's first two cancers were rare liposarcomas, cancers of the fatty tissue.

"Liposarcoma of the vocal cords is extremely rare," Flatow said. "There may be five or eight of these cases in this country. There was deformity, but no recurrence of the cancer."

Ray showed great courage in recovering from the surgery to remove the larynx, Flatow said.

"His speech is remarkable, the best I've ever heard. He communicates beautifully—just did it, and moved his career forward. Then he shows up with a lump in his neck."

At first, doctors felt that lump would be another liposarcoma. Instead, it was a completely separate cancer—a lymphoma that had already reached his bone marrow.

"It was a poorly differentiated, diffuse lymphoma of the back, one of the more rapidly spreading lymphomas. The median survival of patients in his group is a year and a half," Flatow said. "We found the groin and other spots were also involved. We did some studies and found he had this rather generalized tumor.

"I told Ray it had spread all over the body, and he was rather depressed. I sent him to Dana Farber Cancer Institute in Boston, but Ray didn't want chemotherapy. He's more of a naturalist, and felt it might abuse his body. I didn't push the chemotherapy, but I made him get off some pretty crazy food programs and start to eat a good, balanced diet.

"Lo and behold, he started to flourish again. We're 11 years later and he's defied all the odds, kept incredibly active."

Flatow said it is unclear why Ray's disease has reacted so differently from initial expectations.

"It could just be the disease," he said. "Ray doesn't stand alone in that regard. But looking back to 1977, we would have predicted otherwise. I don't know why he's different. I'd have to believe it's life-style and personality, but I can't quantitate that."

Ray's Springfield surgeon, Vincent Guardione, confirmed that he had removed a liposarcoma of the vocal cords and a liposarcoma of the back. He performed surgery for malignant lymph nodes on September 22, 1977, and confirmed the discovery of malignant cells in the bone marrow.

"The course of Ray's lymphoma is extremely unusual," Guardione said, "since he had no treatment for this lymphocytic leukemia, other than eating weeds in Jamaica, or wherever it was and whatever he ate. When you put everything together, the liposarcomas and the lymphoma, it's amazing he's still with us. The current treat-

ment of lymphocytic leukemia, as far as I know, is not 'No treatment.' I'm totally amazed, to be honest with you.

"Of course, he's a pretty unusual guy. For a person to have a laryngectomy, to put in that kind of work to learn esophageal speech, to carry on with his life, he has to be a very determined individual. A never-say-die attitude is extremely important. There are many, many areas of medicine in which science can't explain things. The will to live is so important. I don't have any scientific basis to explain this, but when a patient is as determined as Ray, he or she will overcome things that other people may not be able to overcome."

Bob Bolduc

INTRODUCTION

Bob Bolduc stopped telling his roommate a joke and watched a grave-looking physician cautiously approach his hospital bed.

"This is serious, mister," she warned Bolduc. "You don't have anything to laugh about. You have a grade-four glioblastoma. According to what we know about this tumor, you have about four months to live."

Bob did get serious—but not about making funeral arrangements. Two weeks after his first brain surgery he sat with other cancer patients, listening to a woman explain the cancer support services offered by the Wellness Community.

"If you choose to participate in recovery from cancer, rather than be a hopeless, helpless victim, then you can at least enrich the quality of your life. And you may possibly affect the outcome of your illness," the woman said. "The Wellness Community is not a hospice. It is not a place to come to die."

Bob raised his hand.
"Where do I sign up?" he asked.

Bob's Story

I'm a cancer survivor for whom the metaphor "Wake up and smell the roses" literally came true.

In the 18 months leading up to my cancer diagnosis, I had logged 500,000 air miles, traveling constantly back and forth across the United States, building up my fledgling business. I was on the road two weeks out of every month, and when I was at home I rarely had time to spend with my wife and three kids.

It wasn't the money. I wasn't after money as an end point. I was intoxicated by the success itself, as a definer of my being and a justification for my earthly presence. The money was just a way of keeping score.

I was a winner. Some of the country's biggest corporations were hiring me to train their salesmen. My company, Bold Associates, specialized in teaching "financial selling," how to get senior salesmen to sell to the big executives of a company, the men with the bucks to spend on large computer systems.

My success became my problem. The more successful I was, the more driven I was. And, unbeknownst to me, that drive, spurred on by a deep psychological and spiritual unhappiness, was helping a life-threatening brain tumor to develop.

One morning, I came in from jogging and walked into the bedroom. My wife was sitting, talking with our two daughters and a niece. The pattern on the rug looked strangely fuzzy. I couldn't tell which girl was my daughter and which my niece. I sat down on the floor.

"Guys," I said, "I think I'm going to be sick."

That's the last thing I remember. I know what happened next, though. Linda and the kids told me later. I had a seizure.

An ambulance came, rushing me to the hospital as our teenage son strolled in the door.

I came awake in the hospital emergency room with one of those nozzles of oxygen in my nose. When I told the neurologist about all the headaches I'd been having, he moved me into a hospital room and told me I'd be staying around awhile.

"I'm sorry to do this," he added, "but state law requires me to report you to the motor vehicle bureau. Because you are having seizures, you won't be allowed to drive anymore."

Just like that, in only a few hours, my world turned upside down. Upside down and inside out. I went from high-flying businessman, the fellow on the entrepreneurial fast track, to someone who wasn't even allowed behind the wheel of an automobile. From being an independent businessman who lived by his own wits, to someone who couldn't depend on his own wits to keep him standing upright from moment to moment.

This all seemed bad enough at the time. It's a good thing then that I had no idea what other events were in store just a few days down the road.

My kids and Linda came in to talk with me while I was lying on one of those beds in the emergency room. You know, the kind where you pull curtains around you. But you can still hear everyone else's grief while you're trying to sort out your own. One of my daughters was emotional; the other played it tough. My son was just like me, joking around so he didn't have to look at me directly. Linda was low-profile and very concerned.

That was December 19. Over the next four days I had every test known to man, and a few I think they might have made up on the spur of the moment. The neurologist knew something was there, but he couldn't locate it. Finally, they resorted to MRI—magnetic resonance imaging—one of the most sophisticated diagnostic tools available and, surprisingly, totally painless. Physically painless, that is.

Psychologically, it's another matter. No one explained anything to me about this test. I was told to lie on a slab, and told that I absolutely must not move at all, under any circumstances. Then the slab was pushed into a long, hollow steel cylinder and I lay there while nothing happened. And nothing happened. And nothing happened. It was like being slipped into a burial vault, just the sensation I needed to experience. I concentrated. I didn't move an inch. I meditated on that claustrophobia-producing steel tube.

The MRI provided the answer. Its sophisticated photos showed a tumor inside my skull, in the occipital area of the brain behind my right ear. Home for Christmas, I was in a drugged-up blur. The only thing I remember about that Christmas—the one later predicted to be my last—was that I had hiccups for 48 hours.

Four days later, on December 29, the neurosurgeon removed the tumor. Of course, the big question was the nature of the tumor—benign or malignant. We anxiously awaited the test results.

On December 30, the doctor who first saw me in the hospital emergency room gave me the news: dead within four months. The death sentence was handed down with the authority of medical science, out of the blue, with no warning. Boom. Just like that. At least convicted murderers know the news from the sentencing judge might be bad. Nobody prepared me. I suppose she thought there was merit in blunt honesty. Or maybe she just didn't like my jokes. No one from my family was at my side when she told me. I couldn't tell you what I said. I think I turned numb.

I called Linda. She came over and we had a good cry and held each other and were stunned. I wasn't religious, hadn't been to church in years. But we tried to go to the hospital chapel. Couldn't get in. It was full of people attending a Mass. We waited until Mass was over and everyone left. Then we went in to sit together in peace and quiet.

A nun came into the room, wanting to give me a blessing. In a fit of rudeness, I mercilessly kicked her out. I was beginning to feel an odd, senseless, illogical but unavoidable anger. That anger was to last a long time, and, I believe, helped me find the necessary extra ounce or two of courage.

Even then, on that first day, Linda and I were determined to appeal the death sentence. We just weren't going to give in like that without a fight. We seized on the concept of statistics. The death sentence was based on statistics. Maybe there was a mistake. Maybe there were other statistics. Maybe, maybe, maybe. It wasn't a denial of the diagnosis, but just a prevailing sense that there was more to it than a simple, cut-and-dried "four months left."

The neurosurgeon arrived.

"There was a small tumor, the size of a grape," he said. "We took it all out."

"Does this mean I'm cured?" I asked.

"Well, it's palliative," he answered.

Palliative. I didn't know from palliative. Talk about ambiguity. I tried to get an explanation for the word "palliative" out of him. He just wouldn't go for it, wouldn't take the bite and explain in plain English.

Hiding behind technical jargon. Hedging. I knew the meaning of that maneuver from my professional background. Either he didn't know the meaning of "palliative"—highly unlikely—or he preferred not to discuss its meaning. And I knew what that meant, too. This guy who had just removed this grape-sized, undesirable object from my brain was hoping not to have to tell me the whole truth.

"It's a grade-four glioblastoma," he said. Technical jargon, technical jargon, technical jargon. "But," he added, "I don't know. It just doesn't look exactly right to me."

Linda and I looked at each other.

"Hey," we thought, "they're not sure. Maybe the first doctor was wrong with her four-month death sentence. This is a little different. Maybe we'll be a little different, too."

We seized that hope, relying on it like a prisoner dreaming of a last-minute reprieve. Linda hand-carried the slides of the biopsied brain cancer cells to another lab across the city for a second reading. The results came back: grade-four glioblastoma, but magnocellular variation, very rare.

"This is something unusual. They don't often see this. The tumor is different, and we'll be different," we said. It was grasping at straws, but it gave us something to hope for.

With each passing day, I became more committed to fighting the tumor and more resentful of the sudden loss of independence. I had a lot of anger at the medical community. My doctors were the best in the world, but I was suddenly trapped in this system where people expected me to resign myself to whatever was going on at the moment.

I decided to revolt, to decline the "meek-and-mild-patient" routine. One day I was joking around with my roommate when a woman walked in, dressed in street clothes. Neither I nor my roommate knew her, yet she walked over to my bed and examined my chart.

"Well," she said, "it looks like you're doing well."

"Who the hell are you?" I asked, quite miffed and slightly mystified by such arrogance.

"I'm the chief of nursing for this floor," she answered.

"Well," I responded, "don't you think we're entitled to know who comes into our room?"

She walked out without answering. Clearly, she felt my remark was out of line. But I had decided that health care is a business and I am a paying customer. I—the patient—pay the bills that provide the hospital staff's salary. As such, I expect at least some modicum of respect and consideration. From the hospital's point of view, the doctors are the paying customers who bring in the business. But, to protect my own sanity, I decided to take the stand of a conscious consumer.

Emotionally, I was a basket case. Once out of the hospital, I alternated between periods of consuming, impassioned anger and periods of deep compassion and sympathy for all humanity.

Out walking one day, I saw a car nearly run down an elderly woman. I had livid fantasies of catching the driver and knocking him down. This progressed to being consumed with anger over every wrong ever committed to me during my whole lifetime. I spent hours plotting my revenge, gritting my teeth until they hurt.

On other days, I went around buying homeless people restaurant meals, or being especially concerned about the well-being of a drunk sleeping in a park. In the middle of the most innocuous conversations, I would start crying. Not consciously crying, not sobbing. The tears would just flood my eyes and roll down my cheeks, almost without my knowing.

I kept having this idea of taking off for a weekend in Las Vegas. I hate Vegas. Linda and I do not go there. But I kept thinking, why not just go and throw the dice? Why not see what comes up? Get lost in the shows, the glitter, the laughter, the easy money. I wanted to escape to some kind of fantasy world.

Before my cancer diagnosis, these emotional extremes were disconcerting for me, although I had certainly felt anger, sadness, and compassion in the past. But now, frighteningly, the feelings seemed at times to control me. What did this mean? Who had I become? Was I reacting normally to the incredible stress of cancer? Or was my brain somehow damaged from the tumor or the surgery? Continuing seizures made me wonder if I would ever again feel like a functional human being, let alone one who could drive a car and perform useful work.

Several people had recommended cancer-support services to both Linda and me. As soon as I was able to get around, we attended an introductory meeting at the Wellness Community in Santa Monica. At that first meeting I met others who had received similar "death sentence" diagnoses, including several long-time members who had proved their doctors wrong. That fighting spirit was just what Linda and I wanted. I signed up for an on-going weekly psychotherapy group for cancer patients. Linda joined a separate group for family members.

"Cancer does have perverse benefits," the group leader said at my first meeting. "Are you looking at the positive side, at the enrichment it offers?"

Enrichment? From hearing I would die soon? I didn't know how to react to such a statement. But I had given her authority, granted her teacher status, so I just took in that statement, deciding to adopt it as a challenge.

I listened to others in the group describe the perverse benefits of cancer. And I watched, frequently tearfully, as a woman in the group spent her last days on earth with a dignity, peace, and joy that I would never before have believed possible. I began to understand that there were many levels and textures to life that I, ruled by my achievement-oriented "don't get personal" attitude, had missed. Joys in life had come to others because of cancer, and slowly but surely, I started to recognize and value similar experiences in my own life.

After the surgery Linda and I went down to San Diego to relax. We just walked, meandered around the city, and wandered into a pretty little park. For a while, we sat quietly and watched some children playing. Then we walked through the rose gardens at Balboa, something we hadn't planned to do. That's where the metaphor of taking the time to smell the roses came literally true.

This wasn't the Bob Bolduc that I knew. The old Bob would never have spent an empty, unplanned day wandering around. Who had time to enjoy a bunch of flowers? But now, under the threat of death, I was looking at life.

Before cancer, I had been having trouble communicating with my kids, probably because I was too busy with my own business to really listen to them. During those first weeks and months, when death felt so imminent, I spent many sleepless nights because of medications. I began to use those nights to write letters to my daughters at college, trying to let them know some of the things I was feeling but couldn't talk about.

One day my oldest daughter telephoned. We talked pleasantly and then I passed the phone to my wife. Later, Linda told me what my daughter had said.

"I know Dad's sick," she said hesitantly, "but I like the new Dad better."

For the first time in my life, I began to look critically at that blind drive to achieve that had motivated me for almost 40 of my nearly 50 years. What was it really that I wanted to gain from the incessant flying around the country, the weeks away from my family, the expensive house in Pacific Palisades and the obligations of high-level corporate life?

Linda and I hadn't started out wanting these things. In our 20s, we had dreamed of a small business, of an income comfortable enough to raise a family, of a nice home and good friends. We wanted an all-around, well-balanced life. But it hadn't worked out so smoothly, partly because life isn't smooth, but also partly because I had not been as active and present a father as I should have been.

And now, on top of everything else, I was facing a four-month death sentence.

Oddly enough, I did not at first connect the family problems and the illness with my high-powered life-style. In fact, it had never occurred to me to question that life-style before the cancer appeared. I was pretty much a product of unconscious motivations that began in my own childhood.

My parents were French-Canadian immigrants who came down to New England from Quebec during the Depression. I was born in Hartford, Connecticut, in a section known locally—pejoratively—as Frog Hollow. My parents divorced when I was seven years old, and my father pretty much abandoned me in favor of the bottle. My mother and I moved to Chicopee, Massachusetts, a working-class mill town with serious economic problems. We were poor. But, even worse, I felt the poverty very, very strongly. I always believed we were just one step above the poverty line, a childhood worry which would shape my future life dramatically.

My father had a fourth-grade education, became a lumberjack at 15, rode the rails to Detroit in the early 1930s, and drank like a fish. But he never—never—missed a day of work. The work ethic ruled in those days, along with the hard living, the cold winters, and the shortage of food. My father did not raise me to be happy. When he was around, he taught a life ethic of competition, of fighting hard for the limited winnings.

"Just remember one thing," he used to shout at me in a drunken stupor, shaking a clenched fist high in the air, "you be the best."

The effect on me was twofold. Consciously, I promised myself to be better than my drunken, uneducated father. Unconsciously, I knew I would never be good enough to satisfy him.

I remember my childhood as mostly just me and my mother. We had a big, extended French-Canadian family, of course, but my mother never married again and never had any other children. We skimped. We worried about putting food on the table. I worked my way through high school delivering groceries.

If my father's people were worldly adventurers, my mother's people were stable, united, and very proud. My mother instilled in me a value of family, the value of education, and—again—the drive to excel. This time, the drive was connected to guilt. To make my mother proud, to justify her life, to do right by her family, it was my responsibility to achieve success. And success to our immigrant family meant, clearly, material success.

Education, I decided, was the key to that success. While I was delivering newspapers and groceries in the wealthier sections of town, I realized that the people who lived in those houses had college educations.

When I finished high school, my mother and I left New England for California, where I could take advantage of state-subsidized higher education. I was supporting my mother by working in a factory. At the same time I was earning my two-year Associate of Arts degree.

Armed with that degree, I began my first professional job, as an accounting clerk. I earned my bachelor's degree in accounting in 1963 from UCLA, and went to work for IBM at age 24. I was on my way up. I think of myself as being institutionalized at age 24. At heart, I really wanted my own small business, but my blue-collar background made me feel afraid to try. So instead, I let IBM indoctrinate me.

For the next 20 years or so, I worked in the corporate world, earning successively larger paychecks and promotion after promotion. My model for thought during those years was based on one book, *Think and Grow Rich,* by Napoleon Hill, as I adopted wholeheartedly the American Dream of material success.

But something was wrong. The empty feeling inside me wasn't getting filled. I never found in the corporate world the identity I sought so desperately. Still, I pushed harder and harder, trying to be good enough to ease the ache instilled by my alcoholic father and my second-generation immigrant status.

I went from successful corporate exec to successful entrepreneur, and still I didn't feel I was "the best." Do I think that compulsive drive helped create the tumor? Absolutely. It's not scientific, and most doctors wouldn't agree. But in my heart of hearts, I know the stress of the business and my psychological loneliness helped produce the cancer.

During the last months before diagnosis, I had plenty of clues that my life-style was destructive. My marriage and family were under strain, and my health was obviously deteriorating. I had gained weight from so much living on the road and eating in restaurants, but was still jogging, which created a knee problem. After a knee operation, I set out on a bike, fell and broke my elbow.

One morning, working in my office at home, I started to

feel oddly ill. My stomach suddenly became violently upset. I was dizzy. My head started spinning and I tried to stand up to get to the bathroom. I just went down. I woke up on the floor, with no idea of how long I had been there.

My doctor said it was probably due to the anti-inflammatory medication I was taking for the knee surgery, and I let it go at that. My attitude was that I was invincible, that I had a business and was not able to take time out. Rather than cut back on work, I tried to take on more.

After that, I had two very severe headaches, unusual for me. Once I was in Boston having a posh dinner with a corporate executive, landing a big account. The dinner was cordial but tense, since a lot of money might change hands. Outwardly I was casual, but inside I was very tense over the deal. I started to get a funny, warning feeling inside my head. It developed into a headache covering the whole top of my head. I called it a crewcut headache, because it felt like a crewcut's worth of skull could suddenly explode. Incredibly, I never said a word to the client I was with, finished dinner and the business discussion and drove several hours on the expressway to New Hampshire. I took a couple of aspirin and slept it off. Several months later, in the Midwest during another tense business discussion, the headache happened again. Again I ignored it, took a few aspirin, and waited for relief.

I ignored these headaches, overwhelmingly painful as they were, telling myself . . . Well, I don't know exactly what I told myself. I didn't let myself think about them, and I certainly didn't connect them to either the fainting spell I'd had or my generally deteriorating health. That I ignored these excruciating clues indicates my unwillingness to recognize my critical state.

Several weeks after the second headache came the seizure, the warning that couldn't be ignored.

During those first months of sessions at the Wellness Community, I began to think about all these factors: how my behavior may have contributed to the illness, how my behavior may have resulted from unconscious motives ruling my life, the possibility of change and "perverse benefit" in the face of severe illness.

I also had another, very immediate and more specific issue to consider: treatment. After the initial surgery I needed first to choose the members of my medical team and then to choose the method of treatment. Selecting a medical team was tough, because, once again, we were in unfamiliar territory. Instinctively, I'm a fighter. Linda and I both needed to fight. But that coarse prophecy of my imminent death made us distrust doctors somewhat. How do we find doctors who believed in fighting, who believed the fight could be successful? We were obsessed with statistics. The doctor who could deliver the right statistics would be our doctor.

First, we needed an oncologist, the doctor who would play our team's quarterback position. We arranged an interview with an oncologist recommended through our hospital. In our view, that first meeting was a job interview: Either we hired the guy, or we went on interviewing other candidates.

"Well," he said when we entered his office, "you must be pleased with the additional news, that the tumor is slightly different from most that we've seen."

Hope springs eternal. This guy had focused on our favorite subject, our life raft of sanity. He, too, thought maybe the outcome could be different, the death sentence unwarranted.

"What do you know about this particular variety?" I asked.

"I don't know anything about it," he said. "Let's look it up together."

"Well," I thought, "at least he's got integrity. He's not afraid to say he doesn't know something."

Next we asked about survival statistics.

"I don't give statistics," he said. "I don't talk about odds. I'm here to give treatment."

Far from being annoyed by his abrupt answer, I liked his

no-nonsense approach and his refusal to lay odds on my life. I grasped his optimism as a hook and held on tightly. I could work with him.

We also needed a radiologist. No matter what treatment I chose, it would include radiation. The neurosurgeon had said, "We got the tumor," but no one knew how far the cancer cells might have penetrated the brain tissue. Radiation to eradicate any stray cells is typically the next step.

We visited the recommended radiologist and asked him for odds on my survival.

"When it comes to statistics," he answered warmly, "there's only one that's important: You're either zero or one hundred percent. So let's get to work."

His decision to treat me as an individual case and not as a dot on a graph of cancer-patient statistics felt right to both Linda and me. We hired him, too.

Then came the most crucial decision of the whole deal. A team in San Francisco had had some success in a very risky, still-experimental process, implanting radiation pellets inside the skull. Placing these pellets temporarily near the tumor site, the theory goes, can more effectively destroy any remaining cancer cells while causing less damage to the brain as a whole.

Because of the nature of the brain surgery, I would have to sit in a barber chair and stay awake during the day-long implantation procedure. Then I would have to sit in isolation for six days, with only properly shielded persons allowed to enter my room while my brain cooked. Then the pellets would be removed. And we would wait to see if the whole thing worked.

This decision, with all its ambiguity and uncertainty, was tremendously difficult to make. I am an American businessman, steeped in our "can-do" philosophy. Lee Iacocca, another immigrant's son who lived the American Dream, used to be my hero. The businessman's ethic is to adopt a macho stance: Any problem can be solved with enough information, grit, and determination. So I set out trying to find all the information about the surgery.

But I was stymied. Instead of an obvious choice—the correct choice—the ambiguity remained. I had mounds of information, but no definitive answer. Ultimately I had only my own feelings as a guide. I could just see Iacocca with his board of directors: "Well, fellows, how do you feel about saving this car company? Let's just do what feels right here." I felt incapacitated.

To make this frightening decision I had to learn a whole new set of skills. As a businessman, I relied on a "problem-solving" concept of the world. Give me a task and I'll complete it. Set up a problem and I'll solve it. I learned I couldn't fight for recovery in the same way I could tackle a business problem. You don't do steps one, two, and three and become healed.

I began developing a concept of life as "process." Fighting cancer would be an ongoing process of change and challenge, a lifelong dynamic. I would do everything I could on a day-to-day basis, get some control back in my life when possible, but give up the concept of ultimate control. That belongs not to us, but to a higher power.

My cancer-support group was crucial during the decision-making process. No group member ever told me to have or not to have the surgery. Instead, they shared their own experiences. And I felt easier after hearing that I was not alone. The sharing bolstered my courage. I finally decided the implant surgery felt right for me. I had already started about six weeks of daily radiation therapy, which was surprisingly easy for me. I had no side effects or even tiredness till the end of the whole treatment. The radiation would be followed by the experimental implant radiation, designed to attack possibly cancerous cells more directly than the general radiation. Then, to complete the process, I would have about nine months of chemotherapy.

Linda and I went to San Francisco to visit the hospital where the implants were done. It was a massive institution that

I hated from the moment I walked in the door. Anything that big just can't be efficient. And it wasn't.

We met the surgeon, who reminded me of Alan Alda. We walked into his cubbyhole office, and there was this young guy in an open-necked shirt with his feet planted squarely on top of his desk. He rocked back in his desk chair and remained incredibly casual during the whole discussion, while we talked about cutting into my skull and cooking my brain cells.

I liked the guy.

I began my inquisition, asking for more and more and more information about the procedure and its risks. The risks went up sharply for patients over the age of 50. I was 49.

"You remind me of another businessman patient we had here a few years ago," Alan Alda said, rocking back again. "He was just as demanding as you."

"How's he doing?" I asked the crucial question.

"He's doing great, back running his business down in Birmingham, Alabama."

"I demand his name," I said. "I have to talk to him."

"I'll have to call him first, to get his permission," he said, startled enough by the outburst to take his feet off the desk.

When I talked to the man in Birmingham, he was cautious and conservative, but very friendly. During our several lengthy conversations he never suggested I do the experimental surgery, but told me in detail about his own experience.

In March, fewer than three months after my world turned upside down, I went to San Francisco for the implant surgery. When I went to check in, the hospital had lost my records. Worse still, the night before the surgery they placed me in a ward full of cigarette smokers.

The next morning the surgical team arrived and we began almost immediately. I had a team leader, a nurse who stayed with me at all times. I sat in the barber chair while the surgeon cut into the back of my head. I had local anesthesia, rather than the riskier general anesthesia.

The surgeon needed to place two catheters through the skull and into the brain tissue, for use in inserting the implants. First anesthetic was administered to two small, precalibrated points in the occipital area. Then he drilled into the skull, while I sat there feeling those vibrations of a drill going through my bone. But the worst was when he cut through the protective membrane surrounding the brain.

"Grab my hands and wrists as hard as you can," my nurse said, encouraging me to let the tension out in my hands rather than move my shoulders or head. My nurse watched constantly, monitoring my mental alertness for any problems or oncoming seizures.

The surgeon put the catheters into my head and prepared to drop in the "hot" radiation pellets. That's when everyone leaves. Some doctors in radiation suits come in with the pellets in a lead container, drop them down the chute, and sew me up.

So now I'm literally cooking, emitting radiation out of the back of my head. No one is supposed to be near me now without proper protective gear. Next, it's back down to the radiation department to take another scan, to be sure they got everything in right. At radiation, the line is backed up, so an orderly leaves me outside, in the hospital hall, on a gurney.

Next, another orderly comes along and leaves a nine-month-old baby beside me to await its turn. Here I've gone through this space-age technology, with everything carefully planned and orchestrated for everyone's safety, and some idiot puts a little baby beside my radiating head. I yelled at someone to move the kid away.

After the scan, there's nothing to do but wait. I have my own room where I'm just supposed to hang out and cook for six days, with a lead helmet to wear when anyone comes into the room, so I don't cook them too.

Cooking away with hardly any visitors is a lonely job. Besides hospital staff, only my wife was supposed to come in and out. But one night, after hours, the heavy hospital door slammed open and in stomped my friend Paul, armed with toys and totally unauthorized to be there. When I told him he couldn't stay unless I put on my lead helmet and he put on a lead apron, he told me to lay off. He had come for a very important reason.

For Christmas a year earlier I'd given him a present of my old, smelly running shoes. We have a mutual tradition of totally tasteless gift exchange. So this year Paul returned the old shoes. Only this time, one shoe is automated. It's got wheels and batteries and a little motor, and when I pressed a button, off rolled the shoe, wheeling around the hospital room floor.

The next day, my surgeon came in and told me he was taking a few days off and wouldn't be around to remove the pellets and catheter. I had the strongest, most illogical feelings of betrayal. I tried to call Linda and had a seizure while on the telephone. Linda hung up and called the nurses' station. The nurses scraped me off the floor.

The surgeon had become like a guru, leading me through this whole process. To get through, I had given myself up to him in a way, and I felt so abandoned. I wasn't prepared to accept a substitute guru. To make matters worse, I was walking down the hospital hall the next day, wearing my lead helmet, when this young guy walked past me.

"You're Bolduc," he said. "I'm removing your implants tomorrow."

"Wait," I yelled. "Can I talk to you?"

This boy didn't look old enough to shave. As Milton Berle would say, "I have underwear older than him."

Actually, the whole thing turned out to be child's play. The kid just pulled out a few stitches and slipped the catheter and pellets out of my brain. He did the whole thing in my room in a few minutes.

That was it. He sewed me up and I left the hospital. Linda picked me up and absorbed another of my irrational fits of anger as she drove me back to Los Angeles. I was weak, underweight, with a high white-cell count. No one could tell if I would get better or worse with time, whether the ordeal I had just completed would be effective, whether I would be alive or dead in two or four or six months.

I returned almost immediately to the Wellness Community, which I needed more than ever. Cancer had created a large gap, an immense void in my life that I had no idea how to fill in a positive manner. Those energies that had been channeled into business were still present, mentally if not physically. Yet I could certainly not return to the world of business.

I had to look, for the first time, into a dark chasm of human emotion. For the last three months, my time and energy had been taken up with cancer treatments and terrible decisions. Now I was faced with . . . nothing. Just waiting. When I recovered enough from the surgery I would begin a once-a-month chemotherapy series, but other than that the medical stuff was pretty much over with.

It was devastating. Either I would die or I would face what looked like an empty life. I believed the main task of fatherhood was providing for my wife and children; now I could not do that. Other people were taking care of my clients, and I seemed to have nothing useful to do. There were still major, unresolved hassles with the insurance company and the logistics of maintaining health care. The full reality, the one that doesn't hit while you're in shock from crisis, hits very, very hard in delayed reaction.

I worried about how my illness was affecting Linda and our three children. One daughter wanted to quit college to be with me. The other wanted to know as little as possible about what was going on. My son, at the peak of his teenage years, clearly needed a strong father who could talk, guide, and discipline when necessary. Linda had taken over almost all tasks of child rearing and bill paying and was carrying much too heavy a load.

I was deeply depressed, without knowing exactly what

depression was. Businessmen don't have time to be depressed. But now, unfortunately, I had all of the rest of my life.

For a while, I spent a substantial part of every week participating in Wellness Community activities. Here I obtained the means with which to deal with these problems. In the process, I enriched my life tremendously. This was my haven, my harbor, an integral part of my recovery.

The central activity was still my weekly therapy group, where I began to learn some specific application skills. The peers do all the talking. We laugh a lot. We cry a lot. We bring in any and all emotional issues. I learned that just talking things out can reduce stress. We learned relaxation exercises and visualization techniques, which, I am certain, helped me get through the first set of radiation treatments with absolutely no side effects.

We also learned, by sharing experiences, how to deal successfully with the medical world. The concept at the Wellness Community is to work in concert with your doctor, to take charge diplomatically by making your doctor part of your treatment team. Your team, not his team. This is often interpreted as a sort of hostility toward doctors, but that interpretation is very far from the truth.

I hate nothing more than an unproductive session of doctor bashing. I myself have had excellent medical care. On the other hand, doctors and their personnel make mistakes. Patients need to bring these problems up, but in a positive way. There's a skill in carving out your own space aggressively but not with hostility. When I kept having trouble with some of the secretaries in one doctor's office, I wrote a letter to the doctor, which I first test-marketed in group.

I rewrote the letter many, many times to get the attacking tone out and to make the letter seem helpful and interested. The doctor thanked me for the letter, read it to his partners and tried to institute some of the suggested changes.

I also attended Wellness Community parents' meetings.

Being a parent with three teenaged children and fighting a brain tumor are two jobs that can seem, at times, antithetical. How do you reduce stress in your life and remain a responsible parent? In our parents' group we shared those experiences and tried to find answers to many questions. How much should you tell your children about what's going on? Should you encourage them to know more? How do you deal with knowing you might die, but still maintain a reasonable level of discipline with children? We'd like to think the kids pitch in and help during a life crisis, but the truth is, kids have their own problems, more appropriate to their years.

My favorite Wellness Community activity is the joke fest. Periodically everyone gets together for a potluck dinner and social evening. Your ticket to the celebration is a joke, and the competition for first prize is intense. Some of the jokes are pretty outrageous, involving people with only "two days to live" or a guy with a sexual dysfunction. Outside of a select group of cancer patients, the jokes might seem pretty tasteless.

But actually they're therapeutic. After the first joke fest I attended, which I did not win, by the way, I came away with the victorious feeling of having laughed at the worst crisis of my life. I learned how important laughing is to healing, and especially laughing at yourself. The fellowship of laughter created a team spirit, and the team spirit made my fight for recovery more than a personal battle. Gradually, I stopped pitying myself, stopped feeling like the Job from whom God had taken everything.

During that time I was in the last stage of medical treatment. The chemotherapy seemed almost routine, although I felt uncomfortable sometimes. After about six months of chemotherapy, I had a dream that I shared with my group. I was in the Bronx and needed to go through a very dangerous alley. The alley was filled with rats, animals that I personally fear deeply. But good animals also patrolled the alley. Those good animals annihilated the rats, allowing me to get through.

The dream was so vivid that the message was clear: The

treatments had been successful and I was in remission. The dream told me I was in recovery, and reinforced my courage to ask my doctor if I could discontinue the chemotherapy.

"Pete," I said to my oncologist, "my body is telling me the chemo has done its job. Unless you can give me compelling reasons why we should continue, I want to stop it."

"To be safe, let's take another scan," he replied.

The previous scan had been clean, and this latest one matched up with that. He agreed that we could stop the final few chemotherapy treatments, telling me a few weeks later that I was in remission. The dream, of course, had told me that earlier.

This is the art of diplomatic confrontation, the theory of win-win negotiations in the marketplace. Giving him an option and seeing his needs in concert with mine let us both feel comfortable with the outcome.

In the summer of 1988, more than 18 months after my "four months to live" death sentence, my medical team pronounced me "in remission." I think I'm cured, but the medical people won't use that word for five years. In my heart, in my body, I feel well.

What remains now is the task of living the rest of my life. I can't work again, because I have some disabilities that will probably remain with me the rest of my life: short-term memory loss, body imbalance, hearing impairment, slight tendency to seizures and stuttering. Most of this is brain damage from the surgery or the tumor itself. And although I sometimes yearn for that high-powered life, I know I don't really want to return to my life as it used to be. I've found other ways of measuring self-worth now.

Linda and I are considering alternatives. College tuition is set aside for all three kids, and Linda and I are thinking about ways to scale down our life-style. We may sell our Southern California house and move to Northern California. We may buy some sort of traveling van and spend six months each year seeing the country. We would like to continue to work with cancer patients, helping them come to terms with the most important and vital experience of their lives.

Linda and I have the luxury of time now. We've paid a dear price for it. I wish everyone could have an experience as powerful without having to go through the cancer.

Sharing the cancer experience with others gave me psychological and spiritual tools that, I am certain, were an integral part of my recovery. The more tools, the less stress; the less stress, the greater the chance of recovery. I learned to take control of that which I could. And to leave the rest to God.

EPILOGUE

Bob had a grade-four astrocytoma, a glioblastoma of a very rare variety—a magnocellular astrocytoma, according to his radiation oncologist, Michael L. Steinberg. Steinberg is an associate clinical professor of radiation oncology with the University of California School of Medicine at Los Angeles and codirector of the Santa Monica Cancer Treatment Center.

"The glioblastoma is from the most serious class of tumor a person can get," said Steinberg. "Once considered incurable, untreatable, and insidious, it's a tumor of the supportive cells or connective tissue of the brain. When a biopsy is taken, a pathologist decides if the cells look like astrocytoma. He grades them, deciding how angry or aggressive the cells look. The angriest, most aggressive, are classified grade four. Untreated, statistically the average survival is three months. With radiation, nine months. With radiation and chemotherapy, we might get 12 months.

"The statistic is: Nobody makes it. That's the statistic. But I have a couple of people in my practice who have made it, who have done well. I don't quote statistics be-

cause patients don't need them. I needed something to give Bob some hope, to get him through a very aggressive treatment course.

"I learned real quick that being bluntly honest doesn't get you far in terms of taking care of patients. People want hope—not that you lie to people—but they want to have hope." If there's a time to tell a patient the worst, "it is when things start going to hell—not at the diagnosis. It's cruel to snatch hope away from a patient."

Steinberg recommended the experimental radiation implant procedure, with a special radiation protocol. The general radiation to the brain, as the first phase of treatment after initial surgery, was toned down to decrease risk to brain cells and to inhibit brain necrosis in survivors. The purpose of the next phase, the radiation implant, was to provide a very high dose of radiation to a very small and specific area of the brain where the tumor had been. The risk of causing radiation damage to the total organ is thus lessened, Steinberg said. Finally, the last phase of treatment, chemotherapy, acts as a kind of mopping up of any stray cells that surgery and radiation may have missed.

"We approached Bob with a more aggressive technique—interstitial implant," said Steinberg. "This is not how such patients are normally treated. The treatment approach was substantially aggressive. But Bob was determined that he was going to beat this. He's a very focused, very disciplined guy. Did that help him? I can't quantify that.

"I personally believe attitude can make a difference in how you do, but I don't have the science to prove it. It certainly makes your life a hell of a lot better. A system like Wellness, that imparts that one-day-at-a-time philosophy, is real valuable to the patient.

"The majority of patients would benefit from psychological counseling, but very few have that orientation. It is very important because of the trauma of a cancer diagnosis: looking directly at your mortality. I'm here to bring a patient through the treatment and to cheerlead a little bit. But I can't provide the kind of comprehensive help provided by the Wellness Community."

Bob's neurologist, Gregory Walsh, believes that Bob's rare astrocytoma carries a slightly better overall chance of survival than the most common variety. Bob's illness showed up as a seizure, "because of the tumor-caused irritability of the brain," Walsh said.

Walsh, clinical professor of neurology for UCLA School of Medicine, believes Bob's attitude played a role in his medical care because he took an active role in participating in his own care.

"He's an outstanding guy, energetic and astute. He's the type of guy who has a real positive attitude: 'Here's the problem and how do we approach it?'

"You have to approach each patient depending on how strong they are. Bob's the kind of person who wants to know. And the better educated a patient is, the more they can participate in their own care.

"I deal with seizure patients. You want the least number of seizures possible with the least amount of side effects from the medicine. Some patients don't take it as instructed. If they understand why they're told to do it a particular way, they're more likely to follow through. I can advise what's best, but the choice of whether to do that is theirs."

Effie Fairchild

INTRODUCTION

College recruiter Effie Fairchild was interviewing a prospective student when her doctor telephoned.

"Lung cancer," he said.

Effie hung up the telephone. She finished interviewing the student and finished the two-week recruiting tour. Then she went home to California to find out what the lung cancer diagnosis would mean to her life.

"About six months to two years to live," her doctor predicted.

When Effie told her sister Cindy, they cried. Then they went out and borrowed a lot of money—enough to buy a Biarritz Cadillac, a ritzy car with a shiny steel roof and leather seats, a car built to last a long, long time.

Effie's Story

I've always thought of myself as an adventurer, a pioneer. As long as I have something new to look forward to I know I'll be OK. It's not action and change I fear, but emptiness and routine.

When I was a kid, growing up in Minnesota, I wanted to be a camp director. By the time I was 30, I had achieved that goal and wanted a change. Next, I went to Europe and got paid for it by working in overseas service clubs for U.S. military personnel. My job was planning and leading recreational activities for the guys, like learn-to-ski trips in the Alps and weekend tours of European cities. The job was perfect for me. I was having fun and serving my country at the same time.

I'm one of those patriotic people who tear up and cry like a baby when the flag goes by in a parade. So when the call came to go to Vietnam to open up the first recreation clubs for our fighting men, I figured, "Why not?" I could be of service to people who needed me and to my country.

I packed up my suitcases to go over there and see what I could do. The first Sunday in-country, I planned a coffee call after chapel. Everything was all set, the pastries and the coffee ready for the men, when I looked over into this field and saw the most beautiful wildflowers.

I wanted those flowers for my table. They were the only ones around that hadn't been trampled or ruined by dust and clay. I also noticed some barbed wire, but the wire was lying on the ground, so I didn't worry. I just walked over through the field and picked myself a bouquet.

"Hey, lady," a soldier called from the road. "Do you know where you are?"

"No," I answered.

"You're in a minefield."

I dropped my wildflowers.

"How do I get out?"

"Same way you got in."

I picked up the wildflowers. I wasn't about to leave them. In high heels and a short blue skirt, I tiptoed out of that minefield exactly the same way I had come in.

Then I put the flowers in water, placed them on the table, and served the coffee and doughnuts. It turned out to be a very successful coffee call, the first held for our troops in Vietnam.

I was determined not to be licked by a minefield. I had gone there to do a job, and I intended to do it. I stayed in Vietnam a year. I was a civilian and could have left anytime, but that was the commitment I had made. Twice I worked wearing a gas mask, because Agent Orange gas floated back into our camp. Now I wonder if that had something to do with the lung cancer, but I'll never know for sure.

I wanted to get out of there so bad, but I didn't quit. I was performing national service, helping our men, and so there was no thought of going home without finishing the job. Vietnam taught me a lot about facing death, and about determination and the will to succeed. I never thought I would need those skills to face my own lung cancer, but I'm glad I've got them.

Eventually some other girls came over to help me out, and we opened five service clubs before my term of duty was up. I went home just before the Tet offensive, when I was 33.

After I came home, I spent some time recruiting other girls to go over to run the Vietnam clubs. It was a terrible job to have to do during those years, traveling to college campuses to recruit. But believe it or not, there were some patriotic students even then.

In 1969 I started working toward a doctorate at the University of Oregon. That was the time of all the student riots. Often I was the only one who showed up for class: old patriotic, flag-waving Effie. But I was there because I wanted my degree, not to make a political point.

I wanted to teach, to work with kids, so I wanted to get a doctoral degree in recreation and leisure services. I was good at the teaching, but some of the courses were hard for me. I had a very, very hard time with the statistics course required for my degree. One of my teachers advised me to give up, to quit trying to earn my degree.

"Effie," he said, "you may as well forget it. You'll never pass statistics, and without statistics you can't finish."

That really pissed me off. I was back in the minefield again, determined to pick my way out. I can't stand anyone telling me I can't do something. Determination and enthusiasm count for 99 percent of the successes in this world. I couldn't get up much enthusiasm for statistics, so I doubled my determination.

Despite that professor's prediction, I passed the statistics course. I earned my doctoral degree and became a college professor, teaching leisure and recreation services. From that experience I learned that people in authority aren't always right when they predict the future. They just like to think they're smart and educated and know what will happen.

But nobody knows the future. Nobody knows whether a person walking through a minefield will get blown up or will step out of the field with high heels and skirt intact, to complete the job.

And nobody—except God—knows what will happen to my lung cancer. So I've decided I'm not going to quit before the nine innings are over.

I taught college for many years, but I started to have serious health and respiratory problems and had to quit. Then I left Oregon, went to live with my sister Cindy in California and took a part-time job as a college admissions counselor for the University of Redlands.

Physically I was feeling pretty lousy, and I was depressed, too, because I couldn't do many of the things I enjoyed doing. On May 9, 1987, I stopped smoking.

That's when all hell broke loose. I gained 26 pounds and my ankles and legs became so swollen and uncomfortable I could barely walk. After 41 years, I think, my body had adjusted itself to nicotine, because when I stopped smoking cigarettes I felt worse than ever.

My family doctor took some tests, then called me in for a meeting.

"Gosh, Effie," he said. "I didn't think we'd find all of this."

He sent me to a number of specialists. The edema, they discovered, was the result of "nephrotic syndrome," a kidney disorder that is usually a side effect of some other problem.

An x-ray of the lungs in December, followed up by another in January, showed abnormalities in both lungs. A biopsy revealed "poorly differentiated adenocarcinoma."

That's when the phone call came, at 3:30 in the afternoon, while I was interviewing at the Shiloh Motel in Oregon. I went on to Seattle and had a very successful recruiting trip, interesting a lot of high quality students in the college. I knew I'd have plenty of time to cry later, but I had a job to do. It was really important for me to do my best.

On February 19, I went alone to see the oncologist, to hear the news and sort it out. I remember two things he said: that the cancer was inoperable because it was in both lungs, and that radiation wasn't a possibility.

I asked for the prognosis.

"It's not good," he said. "Six months to two years."

He suggested either chemotherapy or experimental treatment.

At the doctor's office, I didn't react too much to his statements. But when I got home, the reaction hit pretty hard. Before I went to Vietnam, I had watched my mother die from lung cancer. My mother, too, had been given six months to two years to live. She made it through 18 months, but they were awful months. There was no quality of life for her. Almost immediately after her diagnosis she went downhill, living with considerable pain, barely able to walk or to function, taking a lot of pain killers like morphine. I watched her waste away to

65 pounds. So I started off feeling hopeless—six months to two years.

"This is exactly the same as Mother," I thought to myself. "I'm going to follow in her footsteps and die in the same way."

I'm not a hopeless, negative person. But with the image of my mother's illness so clear in my mind, I thought I knew what the future held. Finding hope, finding the energy to fight became a daily struggle. I may have walked out of that minefield, and I may have passed that statistics course, but I just wasn't prepared to fight for my life against the very thing that had taken my own mother.

Every night I put myself to sleep going over the diagnosis from the doctor. It was cancer, cancer, cancer all the time. Every waking minute, and even in my dreams, my mind was dominated by illness and death. I didn't sleep much and when I did, my dreams were of cancer. Mornings, I lay in bed until 10:00 or 10:30, not wanting to get up, feeling I had nothing to get up for.

My sister took over responsibility for everything. She had power of attorney and handled my business affairs, ran the household, and made sure I kept my appointments and took my medication. I just gave up. All I could see was my mother, wasting away. I was waiting for that to happen to me.

But there was something else happening too. At the doctor's office I had picked up some papers about some cancer support groups. I had conflicting feelings about attending a group, because I had always handled things by myself.

While I was thinking over what I wanted to do, the woman running the group met me in the doctor's office. It was after my first chemotherapy treatment, and I was feeling lousy.

"There's a group you can attend," she told me softly. "You don't have to do this alone."

She gave me a list of books to read, and told me more about the Wednesday night cancer group. She offered some advice, and left. My barriers went up immediately.

"I can handle this myself," I thought, while driving home from the doctor's, ignoring the fact that obviously I was not handling the cancer very well. But I had always been in charge of my life, and I thought attending a group would be giving over control, admitting weakness.

I figured a cancer group would be a lot of people sitting around whining and complaining and feeling sorry for themselves, and I didn't need that. I figured a support group would be like going to a shrink. I had known friends who had gone to shrinks, and I knew I would never need to do something like that.

But at the same time I was thinking that maybe it was time I stopped fighting the battles by myself, maybe it was time to call in some reinforcements. I had always been a general or a sergeant major. Maybe now it was time for me to be a private.

I used to teach my students to follow the "Celestial C's" when organizing community service programs: Cooperation, Collaboration, Communication. I taught them to cooperate and share—good advice. But I hadn't followed that advice in my own private life.

"Maybe I should apply these teachings," I thought. It certainly couldn't hurt, because I couldn't make myself more miserable than I already was.

While I was thinking this over, I was having chemotherapy treatments. Those treatments just drained me of every last ounce of energy.

"It's not like a truck has run over me," I told Cindy. "It's like the truck is sitting on my body and won't ever get off."

I even had to call for help on my job, because I couldn't find any more energy for college recruiting. That admission was difficult.

I decided to go to group, to try just once. I kept thinking of the group leader, Shannon McGowan, saying softly, "There's a group you can attend." Cindy agreed to come, too, as a support person.

I was so afraid the group would be emotional, and I wasn't ready for a lot of emotion about cancer. But I went anyway. I was one of the first people there. And when Shannon came in, she didn't remember me. I felt awfully alone, and wanted to get up and run out.

Everyone sat in a circle, and Shannon asked someone to talk. After a few others spoke, she asked me to say something. There's a box of Kleenex at all these damn things. I looked at that box.

"Oh, God, Effie, you're going to lose it," I thought.

I just started crying. At one point, I couldn't breathe. I just couldn't find any courage, and cried like a baby.

While I was crying, a man walked in who was a recovered alcoholic. He started telling me that he had also been successful in dealing with his lung cancer. He gave me so much hope, because he could tell his story without crying. We gave each other a hug.

He pulled a black poker chip from his pocket—the acknowledgment of his nine years of sobriety—and handed it to me. That chip went straight into my wallet, and has been there ever since. It's filled with luck, and the luck has rubbed off on me on more than one occasion.

That chip and that hug and that first group meeting helped turn me around. I began to get a grip again and began to find some fighting energy.

The group presented me with the three H's every cancer patient needs: Hope, Humor, Healing. The "hope" you've already seen—someone who had been through my illness and could talk about it.

Every meeting is filled with humor, along with some tears, too. Anyone coming in off the street would have a hard time believing we are cancer patients because we laugh so much. But we do laugh about some pretty bizarre things. When I was taking chemotherapy my brother sent me a green wig, which I wore to the support group one night.

"Look what happens when your hair grows back," I warned everyone.

They thought the joke was pretty funny. But when I pulled that trick in a cancer-education group, "I Can Cope," people sat in shocked silence.

"How can she make fun of something so serious and dreadful?" one woman asked a friend of mine.

I made fun of the baldness because I think you can be healed through humor and laughter. In our support group we make life a game. Sometimes you have innings when you're down and out, and sometimes you're a winner.

The "healing" in the group came from many sources. Most of my friends had called or written letters or visited when they heard about the cancer. But there were three people who just didn't call or write or do anything. I had thought they were close friends, but they wouldn't acknowledge my cancer and had just written me off.

I was really pissed. My anger was causing me a lot of stress, which I didn't need to add to my life, so I told the group.

"Why don't you write them a letter," someone suggested. "Get rid of the stress, and give it to them. Let them handle it."

So I wrote three piss letters.

"I'm really surprised that you haven't acknowledged my illness," I wrote. "I have cancer and I'm fighting it. I wonder why I haven't heard from you."

I signed the letters "stress-freely yours."

All three answered. One woman wrote back, another called, and the third sent a long letter, followed by weekly postcards.

That's part of healing, getting rid of all the excess baggage that gets in the way of living. In group we talked about taking positive actions, like buying the Cadillac, about changing lifestyles and trying new things. We talked about setting goals and looking forward to experiences in the future.

Still, there were times when I didn't want to go to group.

Some people in remission who had left group came back with recurrences, which discouraged me. I told Cindy I might quit.

"Fine," she said. "Do what you want. But I'm still going."

"What the hell," I thought. "If my own sister's going, I may as well go too."

I was fighting, trying to believe I would get better, but deep down inside I didn't believe I would. I just kept remembering my mother and hearing "six months to two years."

During April and May I got more and more depressed. Despite the group, despite the Cadillac and the green wig, I felt myself gradually losing the will to live. Losing my hair was so degrading. And I had so little energy.

Inwardly I wondered if life was worth the trouble. I kept thinking of that Peggy Lee song, "Is That All There Is."

"Effie," I thought to myself, "you've had a good life. Maybe this is a good time."

Death frightened me, but I figured I could handle it better than the life I thought was in store for me.

"Let's just get it over with before it gets worse," I thought. But I couldn't say this to anyone. To my friends I was "one tough lady," so outwardly I put on that facade.

Once I visited Shannon, the support group leader, alone.

"I think I'm giving up," I told her.

I expected her to say "Oh, God, Effie. Don't do that." Instead she asked me to talk about how I was feeling. She didn't try to change my mind. She just listened, and helped me feel OK about these thoughts. We did some relaxation exercises and some mental imagery. Talking to Shannon helped ease my guilt about maybe wanting to die, and it helped me understand that sharing isn't a weakness, but a strength, a strength that comes from numbers.

Still, I just couldn't rid myself of the brooding and dread I felt. Then, in July, everything came to a head. A friend was visiting, and we were swimming in the pool. I was showing off, swimming laps under water while holding my breath, just to prove that I was still the same old Effie.

I developed an incredible headache, a "steel" headache, the kind that feels like a piece of steel hitting me over the head again and again and again. There was this heavy steel feeling all over the top of my head. I had called my doctor, who told me to watch it, and call him the next day if the pain continued.

Tuesday morning I called him back, and he said to make an appointment for a brain scan. So I got out the phone book and started searching for the phone number. I could read the name of the business, but when I tried to read the phone number, I couldn't see the whole number at one time. I could read the first group of numbers or the last group of numbers, but I couldn't read all seven at once.

I called Cindy, who was at work.

"I can't see," I told her. "I can't do anything. I just want to go to the hospital."

I had never, never volunteered to go to the hospital before. Cindy realized I was seriously ill and came home immediately. We went to the doctor's office.

"I can't see you," I told the doctor. "I'm seeing blurs."

I answered some questions they asked me, but by this time I was no longer conscious. I don't remember anything that happened to me for the next three days, although clearly my mind was registering events around me on an unconscious level. When people asked me questions, I answered them, but the answers were nonsensical and sometimes not even in English.

I spent the next two days in the intensive care unit, wired to monitors, staring out at the world with glassy eyes. A spinal tap showed blood in the spine, an indication of a brain hemorrhage. Tests showed something that could have been a clot in the brain, or possibly a tumor.

The doctor told Cindy I was deteriorating and that it was

time to call the family around the country and let them know I was dying. Cindy spent two days calling family and friends.

In the ICU, while I was emotionless, blind, glassy-eyed, and speechless, the doctor's message about my impending death somehow reached my subconscious level.

I decided not to die. I can't explain what I mean by that, except that my subconscious didn't like the idea of me deteriorating.

On the third day, I started seeing things and talking again. Most of what I said was gibberish, and I saw some rather odd things. Everyone who came into my room had black eyes, mustaches, green coats, and disabled arms.

But I knew who people were.

"Do you know who I am?" my doctor asked.

"Of course," I said. "You're Doctor Igdaloff. Sometimes I call you Iggy."

I don't think he appreciated that. The woman doctor whom I accused of having a mustache wasn't laughing either, but eventually my brain straightened out even these minor misconceptions.

No one ever pinpointed what did happen in my brain during those days. After two CT scans, three MRI scans, numerous blood tests, two spinal taps, and eight full days in the hospital, at a cost of $13,000, the doctors scratched their heads and said it was a puzzle. No cancer cells were located anywhere in the brain.

Gradually, I returned to my old prehospital self. Except that I had changed in one essential way. The terrible depression disappeared. While I was in the hospital, so close to death during those two days, I felt a serenity and a marvelous feeling of letting go.

It's OK to let go, I realized. Death is not to be feared, if this is what it's like. And when I stopped fearing death, I could start living again.

I also realized that the course of my illness will be mine

and mine alone. I am not my mother, and I will not have to follow in her footsteps.

With that realization, I could begin to hope again. And with the return of my hope came the return of my enthusiasm for life. Instead of staying in bed, planning for my death, I began to look forward to new experiences and I began to feel again that I had something to offer the world.

The luck of that black poker chip tucked away in my wallet carried me through the hospital, and it carried me on to a winner's streak in life.

Several weeks after my hospital episode, Cindy and I and Ardis, my ex-nun buddy, headed the old Cadillac up to Reno to see what the slot machines held in store. I pulled down three jokers and waited while 1,977 nickels cascaded down, enough to fill two large buckets. After that, we headed over to the Indian reservation, and I won $2,000 at bingo in one night.

Cindy and Ardis and I went back to Reno to see the Smothers Brothers. I think their laughter is very healing for me. While we were in Reno, I drew an ace, queen, and 10 of hearts on the progressive nickel machine.

"Cindy," I said, "I'm going for the big one. I know I can do it."

"You'll never get it," she answered. "No one ever gets a royal flush on these things."

I thought about that. I thought about getting out of the minefield. I thought about passing the statistics course. I thought about getting out of that intensive care ward.

And I remembered the big lesson I had learned. No one ever knows for sure what's possible in this world. I threw away the two useless cards and kept the three hearts.

I drew two other cards. The king and jack of hearts came up. Out of the machine poured $268 in change.

I've been feeling like a winner ever since the hospital. And when you feel like a winner, you are a winner.

As my strength returned, I wanted to do more physically

active things, but I still couldn't play much tennis or swim for too long. A friend brought up yoga. Yoga, she said, could be very strenuous or very relaxing, whatever is appropriate.

I had in mind the Jane Fonda workout stuff, with the fancy outfits and the jumping around. Either that, or strange people sitting cross-legged chanting for hours in a weird language. "Thanks," I said. "But I don't think so. It's a little too far out for me."

But she insisted. When I went, I was mesmerized. The teacher was a pleasant, warm woman dressed in a Peking sweatsuit, barefoot, with a soft voice.

"If it hurts, don't do it," she said. I found that yoga was a gentle activity, relaxing and noncompetitive. After the first class I felt calmer than I had in weeks.

And when my yoga teacher took a lengthy trip, I took over her early morning bread run. Three mornings a week now I rise at 6 a.m. and head down to the local supermarket. I stuff the day-old bread into the car and drive down the freeway, over the bridge into San Francisco. The bread goes to a soup kitchen run by Mother Theresa's sisters. There are hungry people in the world and I can help. Some people are down and out in the world for no reason we can understand. Maybe this will be the meal that gets them going. And I'm so glad I have the privilege of helping.

I'm also busy two or three days a week helping to begin a Northern California branch of the Wellness Community, started down in Santa Monica. This has become my new pioneering effort. The philosophy of the community is to provide free, continuous support to cancer patients. My own cancer support group helped so much, but it's very difficult for a cancer patient in crisis to wait until 7 o'clock Wednesday night to talk. A cancer patient needs to get help any day of the week, at any hour of the day. That's the kind of help the Wellness Community provides.

I don't do any of these service jobs full time, because I'm

trying to balance my life and keep it stress free. Sometimes now, when I don't feel like doing anything at all, I go down to an expensive haircut place and get my hair done. Or I take a bath, using the French bubble bath I bought myself a few weeks ago. Or I go out and take pictures of pretty scenery. I never did any of this before I went into the hospital.

Some people have trouble thinking I have lung cancer. The other day at yoga I was talking about my bread run to a friend in yoga class.

"You're having so much fun in life, Effie," she said. "How do you do it?"

"I have to have fun," I told her. "I have lung cancer, and having fun is part of my healing."

She was shocked that I had such a serious illness.

Medically, they might say there is no reason for me to live. But psychologically, there are many reasons to live: my bread run, the new Wellness Community, my yoga, and—most importantly—my family and friends.

For the past 14 months I've maintained an excellent quality of life, despite the brain problem that took me into the hospital. My cancer has stabilized, with no change since diagnosis. And I hope to maintain that quality of life for another five or ten years.

I don't think this is "false hope." I just think a person's attitude has a lot to do with health. The figures on lung cancer are 15 and 85. That is, 15 percent are winners. So if we're going to play the numbers game, I'm going to play the winning odds.

EPILOGUE

Effie's oncologist, David M. Igdaloff of Walnut Creek, California, said Effie's disease seems to have arrested. The tumor in the lung remains basically unchanged 14 months after diagnosis.

Igdaloff said he could not explain the cause of the neurological problem that brought Effie into the hospital.

"It was some type of acute vascular event," he said. "But there was no evidence of tumor in the brain; the specific cause was never determined. We expected her to die. She deteriorated very rapidly right in front of our eyes. She had high blood pressure and abnormalities in the brain according to the scan. Then she got better. We kept thinking a tumor would show up in the brain, but it never did. It was almost a miracle."

Igdaloff supports the idea of a cancer support center.

"We [physicians] can treat the physical elements, but we don't have the expertise and time to give the psychosocial support. I haven't done a formal analysis, but patients who do use these services report they have benefited."

Bonnie Hopkinson

INTRODUCTION

At 41, Bonnie Hopkinson was disappointed with life. She had so much—a husband of 20 years, a handsome teenaged son, a pleasant Toronto home by the shore of Lake Ontario. Yet she felt empty, starved for love and meaning in life. She lived with a constantly gnawing feeling that she would never be loved because she was not worth loving.

When Bonnie was diagnosed with breast cancer, she looked deeply for the first time at that loneliness. She found, buried deep in her subconscious, the reason for her sadness. And she found a group of people who helped her better understand the nature of love.

Bonnie's Story

Getting cancer was a call for love. I had never had a good self-image throughout my life, and I was never confident that I was liked or loved by others. My husband and son loved me, of course, but that somehow never seemed real to me.

When I got cancer, I thought of it as a challenge, to show everybody how strong I was and to thereby get their love. But I was to learn that I wasn't calling for the love of others, but calling for love within myself.

I'm not talking about self-love as a conceit, about how pretty I am or how smart I am. I'm talking about self-love as love for everything that I am, accepting myself for the things I'm good at. And for the things that I'm not good at.

All my life I had been caught up in meeting the expectations of others, in being a good wife to my husband, a good mother to my son, a good secretary to my boss. It's not that people put those expectations on me; it was how I believed people expected me to act. There's a big difference in those few little words.

Despite my struggle to meet those supposed expectations, I always felt like a failure. I always felt undefined. I needed to find out that it was OK to be me. Without having a big career to say who I am. Or a big house to say who I am. Or a large family to say who I am. Or an artistic life. I needed to accept just being me, without any symbols declaring my right to be on this earth.

When I was 21, I married my Michael, my high school sweetheart. By that time, I had already been working as a legal secretary for four years, at a job I started right out of high school. I had wanted to be a veterinarian, but that was for intelligent people. My aunt was a secretary, and when she suggested I specialize in some area of secretarial work, I picked law. It seemed as interesting as anything else, and I would earn a decent living.

I worked for 10 years for the same man, and I enjoyed it. I felt good about doing some useful work. Then, when I had my son, Matt, I decided to stay at home instead of returning to an office. I thought if I could relax and enjoy being a mother, I would be able to have another child. But it didn't happen. And I began to be restless, just being at home.

Then began a difficult time, stretching through most of my 30s. I tried so hard to find something "to be." I wasn't really a mother, you see, since I only had one child. When people asked how many children I had, I never said, "One." I always said, "Just one." I hadn't produced enough, and I felt that made me a failure at motherhood.

I tried returning to work as a legal secretary, but found I couldn't do it anymore. The work that had given me so much pride as a young woman now left me with an empty and unfulfilled feeling. I went through sporadic starts and stops, looking for some kind of direction, hoping that something would give me the feeling of validity in my life. I tried learning crafts, working in shops, taking university courses. Nothing worked.

In 1982, my husband got a job in Connecticut. This was the first time I had ever lived more than 10 miles from the city of Toronto. Secretly, I was ecstatic to be away from all the people who thought of me as "nice little Bonnie." I could do whatever I wanted to do, be whoever I wanted to be, without worrying about what everyone else would think. I did some volunteer work with the Connecticut Audubon Society and found that I loved being part of the world of nature. I felt I was beginning to achieve some independence and individuality.

Three years later, we came back to Toronto. I fell back into the old mold again, as layer upon layer of my old life fell on top of me, covering me over again. I began to fulfill old expected roles, and the new ones, developed in Connecticut, dissolved. I couldn't even continue my learning about nature, because the natural world just doesn't exist in Toronto.

I gave in. I decided to quit fooling around, to stop all the nonsense of "finding yourself." There was nothing to find, I decided, nothing there besides "nice little Bonnie."

We needed to make some money, so I decided to go back into an office to work, after taking a computer literacy course to bring me up to date. All through the fall of 1985, while I was learning about computers, something was nagging inside me. I just had the feeling I wasn't doing the thing I was supposed to be doing. I felt like I was going against myself.

"What are you doing?" this tiny voice kept whispering. "You don't want to go back into an office."

In November 1986, about a year after I decided to return to the office work, I was diagnosed as having breast cancer. The physical growth inside my body was a symbol of the emotional and spiritual growth that I needed, but kept denying. There were so many urges in me to do things, and I didn't do them. I think my spirit was slowly dying. My inner self was dying, getting ready to leave this body because it didn't have a chance to manifest itself.

I felt that the cancer gave me permission, for the first time in my life, to follow my own inner voice, to explore my own interests. I felt people would be saying, "Oh, she has cancer now. She can do anything she wants."

Actually that was me, finally giving myself permission to follow my own inner voice. I started by joining a cancer-support group, where I learned meditation and visualization and where I could explore ideas with others who were thinking about the same things.

I also began pursuing my interest in yoga. For the longest time I had had a secret interest in yoga, but hadn't told anyone about it. Learning yoga would have made me a real oddball and I wanted people to like me. Before cancer I wouldn't take any small steps out of the mold in which I thought people had placed me.

The first small lump was surgically removed, but in October 1987 I had my first recurrence, and yet another in February 1988. I felt this second recurrence was a nudge from my body, telling me to pay more attention to the inner emptiness I always had felt.

I knew there were feelings buried deep down inside me,

feelings of anger and grief that I never felt or expressed, feelings that seemingly had no source I could pinpoint. On the surface I continued to live my life as "sweet little Bonnie."

Michael and I together decided I would go alone to a yoga retreat in western Massachusetts. I had never done anything like this before. I wanted to, but it seemed selfish to take money the family needed and spend it on myself.

"Go ahead," Michael said. "Go. Do whatever you need to do."

We made this decision on faith. I didn't know anything about the ashram, about the kind of people there. Michael wasn't sure I wouldn't come back with my head shaved, wearing orange robes. I didn't know that either but I took the chance.

Being alone in a strange place, talking to men I didn't know, was a new experience for me. I had been lifted out of my lifelong cocoon and put down in a new world. Besides yoga, we had many other exercises. We practiced circle breathing, which creates a special kind of energy called "prana."

During one of the exercises, I visualized my father coming toward me, telling me that he loved me. I hadn't known my father when I was a child. He was an alcoholic, and my mother sent me away to live with relatives so that my father wouldn't harm me.

I saw my father coming toward me, telling me that he loved me very much and that he was sorry he hadn't been able to be a father to me. I felt all the grief and sadness and loneliness and emptiness coming together in one rush of feeling and I finally understood that I wasn't the cause of my father's actions and that I was, after all, truly loved by him.

I never even knew I had missed having a father. I never knew that all my sadness had come from that loss of love, buried so deeply so long ago. Later on, during a breathing exercise, I felt a special, strong sort of energy that made me feel so vibrant that I started to roar with laughter.

"Your eyes are so bright," someone said to me. "You're shining and radiant. You look so changed."

I felt changed. Something in me had shifted finally. At the end of the retreat, those who wanted stood in front of the group and spoke to everyone. I listened while a man told about the guilt he felt after fighting in Vietnam.

"OK," I thought. "I can do this."

I stood in front of everyone and began talking.

"I admire you all so much," I told them. "You are willing to learn about life before you become ill. I am here now because I am a cancer patient. And I am so glad to be here, to have learned what I have learned here. My only fear is that I will die before I find out who I am."

Never before had I dared speak to a group like this. As they gave me a standing ovation, I felt another surge of energy and a new confidence in myself. I felt healed.

There is a difference between healing and curing, a difference that is somewhat subtle but very important. A healing is an experience of the soul. A cure is the cessation of illness. I don't know what will happen to my illness. The cancer may or may not be cured.

But the sadness in my soul has begun to heal. At the ashram I felt surrounded by many supportive and loving men and women. I felt safe and I felt able to face my sadness. What I experienced there—the vision of my father walking toward me—filled me with a new understanding of my life, and of the lives of my mother and my father. That mysterious, aching emptiness was finally filled with the knowledge of love.

This healing, which I may not have experienced without the cancer, has given me new strength, courage, and confidence.

EPILOGUE

Bonnie has had a somewhat atypical breast cancer, a lumpectomy, and then a recurrence locally, according to her oncologist, Robert Myers, of Toronto's St. Michael's Hospital. After the initial diagnosis, preventive chemotherapy was recommended.

"She's a patient who has strong views on what her treatment should be, and she wasn't too keen on starting the chemotherapy treatment immediately," said Myers. "She's been very interested in pursuing all avenues, so it wasn't unusual for her to be referred to a cancer support group."

Myers does not believe the support group has affected her physical health.

"I don't think this affects health at all, but that's just my opinion. There's a certain type of person who will benefit from group sessions, one who is introspective and intelligent, but these people are certainly not representative of cancer patients in general. In terms of making people live longer, I doubt it. But if it makes people feel better, then fine. The main thing is to help people make good use of their time."

Lisa Whiteside

INTRODUCTION

One fall day Lisa Whiteside strapped a rhinestone cat collar around her neck, flipped an uncomfortable wig off her bald head, and marched down Boston's elegant Newbury Street, past galleries, boutiques, and cafés. Passersby stared as she and her soberly dressed sister-in-law played out their outrageous street theater: New England matron interviews prospective punked-out California nanny.

Bald from five months of chemotherapy prescribed after a recurrence of ovarian cancer, Lisa was discouraged, depressed, and angry. She still had the cancer, which had failed to respond to the chemotherapy, only now she had no hair. Her baldness symbolized her separateness from other young women—her cancer.

Lisa fought her depression using her favorite weapon: the practical joke. She flaunted her baldness down Newbury Street, self-conscious yet laughing all the way.

That winter, Lisa sent Christmas cards with a photo insert. Wishing everyone a Merry Christmas was a grinning Lisa—bald head, cat collar, and all.

Lisa's Story

I intend to live—to be truly alive, that is—until I die. In many ways—despite the progressive cancer and the radiation and chemicals used to treat it, despite the fear from facing death—I am more alive today than I was that February day in 1980 when the doctors walked into my hospital room to give me the bad news.

Along with the surgeon were two resident physicians and three medical students. The whole crew circled my bed, and the surgeon, obviously uncomfortable, spoke.

"We found a tumor," he said. "It was malignant."

Shocked, barely comprehending, I pulled the covers over my head. That was my habitual response to crisis: avoidance.

But with cancer, denial doesn't work. I had to learn that, for me, hiding from the truth does much more harm than good. Some people just close the doors and the shutters on life. But that's by choice, not necessity. At this moment, my prognosis is uncertain. I've been told I won't survive this disease. But I've also been told I could live a long time with the disease.

Before my diagnosis, I was helping the director of development raise funds for a Boston area college. I wasn't stimulated by my job, didn't feel like looking for anything else, dated a man casually in a "no commitments" relationship, and lived in an apartment I didn't particularly like. Mostly, I remember the apartment, a dingy fourth-floor place with a window looking out on the wall of another dingy apartment building.

That window barely let in the light of day, but it didn't matter too much. The light elsewhere in my life was minimal, too. I lived in an eternal low-key depression, thinking about changing everything in my life but never acting on it.

Physically, I felt tired but never suspected any kind of serious illness. I attributed my feelings to my emotional outlook. However, I did finally go to see my internist because of a lingering cold.

"By the way," I told him, "I feel this lump sometimes."

He ordered lots of tests. When I went down to the lab in the basement of the same building, the technicians kept taking more and more pictures.

"Great," I thought. "They've got all this equipment and they need to make some money from it, so now they've got an excuse to charge the insurance company and rake it in."

Another doctor had told me not to worry about the lump, and I was trying to avoid being labeled a hypochondriac. Now, with this guy ordering tests, I stayed skeptical. I had no blockage or nausea or any kind of discomfort—just this lump. Who thinks about cancer, especially ovarian cancer, at 31?

The tests showed a definite solid mass in the middle of my abdomen. Surgery, the internist advised. The internist referred me to a surgeon, who felt little sense of urgency, allowing me to choose an appointment totally at my convenience, based on the pressures of my office responsibilities. No one ever spoke the word "cancer."

"The feeling is," the doctors agreed before surgery, "the lump will probably be benign."

During the surgery, the medical team agreed that the lump appeared to be malignant, but they kept this from me until the final pathology report came in.

They told my therapist, who came to see me soon after surgery. He had worked with me for two years by then and was a source of strength and caring in my life. His visit to the hospital supported me when I was so frightened.

The doctors also told my parents about the malignancy while I lay there, supposedly recovering and thinking everything was fine. I learned later, from another doctor, the details of what happened while I was under anesthesia: When he uncovered the lump, the surgeon said sadly, "It looks bad."

Being kept in the dark upset me. I wanted to be part of the team, not soothed and protected from the truth.

After the doctors came to tell me about the malignancy, I felt almost guilty.

"Why is this happening?" I asked myself over and over and over. "What have I done to create this?"

While I was going through this agony of self-recrimination, one doctor returned.

"I just wanted you to know," he told me softly, "there was nothing you did to cause this disease, and there was nothing you could have done to prevent it."

Those few words lightened my burden. Coming at such an intense moment—right after the diagnosis—they remain vivid and vital to this day. Cancer patients bathe in guilt, sometimes exacerbated by poorly explained "holistic" ideas. I had heard bits and pieces of this philosophy, and I interpreted the concept of "responsibility" for illness in a very personal and literal way. To me, being "responsible" for my illness meant I secretly, unconsciously, wanted cancer and maybe even wanted to die.

A cancer diagnosis requires psychological as well as physical energy. The burden of such guilt only adds weight to a load that already seems unbearable. This young resident, a future plastic surgeon and adept interpreter of medical details, recognized my self-made trap and helped loosen it.

The tumor had grown in a very unusual way. It was self-contained, meaning it apparently hadn't spread elsewhere in the abdomen. But it had wrapped around the intestine. The tumor was low-grade, slow-growing, and less aggressive than most. Despite the tumor's clearly ovarian origin, the ovaries themselves contained only microscopic disease.

Because of the extensive cancer, the surgeon advised a complete hysterectomy. I was to go home and recuperate physically for six weeks. After the hysterectomy I would have six weeks of radiation treatments. The whole process would require about five months.

Trusting the doctors' statement that a deadly disease had invaded my body required an act of faith. I had no unbearable aches and pains, no debilitating fevers, no paralyzed limbs. My body was the same as always.

Still, I wanted the cancer out of my body. Out-of-control cells were running loose in my body, and I started to feel out of control thinking about that. Throughout the interminable six-week wait, I tried to reconcile the conflicting feelings. I couldn't face the hysterectomy—losing, at 31, the chance to have children—but I wanted the cancer out of there. I was in a holding pattern, neither alive nor dead, waiting to get rid of these deadly cells.

At home, by myself in that apartment, I felt alone in a deep, dark, intangible way. In the early morning hours, in that apartment with that dingy window that looked out onto that dingy wall, the night terrors came. In the dark, alone, I imagined terrible, insurmountable horrors—pain, long-term debilitation—and wondered desperately how I would ever cope. At the hospital, the 24-hour nursing staff had helped allay those terrors. Alone at home, I lived on a roller coaster of emotions that wouldn't let up, that focused on the disease running rampant inside my body.

Depression, previously low-keyed, took center stage, ruling my life. There were very dark times. Was it worth it? I couldn't shake the dark aspects and even thought about suicide.

My imagination was my own worst enemy. I had little experience with illness, with pain, or with spiritual resources. I imagined the worst, more on the basis of hysteria than a real understanding of cancer. No one really talked about cancer, so how could I have known the truth about my illness? Massive, unbearable pain surely lay ahead, I convinced myself. "If I'm going to be in terminal pain," I thought, "I would just as soon check out. I don't want that, and I don't want to be debilitated, living on life-support systems. If it comes to that," I decided, "I can commit suicide."

Unspoken conversational taboos worsened my isolation. Friends and family loved and wanted to help me, but we became locked in a sort of overprotective dance: They didn't want to upset me by bringing up the cancer, the matter we needed most to talk about. In turn, I thought, "Oh, I can't bring it up with them. They're already so uncomfortable."

But when I did start discussing the cancer, people responded. Talking about the diagnosis with friends helped lessen my feelings of isolation, at least taking the cancer out of the realm of "the unspeakable." Incredible amounts of love were directed toward me. Friends expressed essential feelings for the first time: "We care about you." "We love you and are scared for you." "We don't want you to die."

The surgical team performed the hysterectomy, intended to remove any cancer left in my body, in April 1980. In the hospital right before the surgery, losing my ability to bear children felt overwhelming.

"I think you can beat this," my primary surgeon was saying.

But I hadn't the heart to feel enthusiastic. Along with the loss of my chance at motherhood came the fairly discouraging statistics for survival with ovarian cancer. I was driving myself crazy reading those statistics. All the numbers, all the prognoses I could find in the library, lodged front and center in my mind. Eventually I gave up the numbers game. Numbers don't reflect individual variation, so reading numbers incessantly only lessens my own individuality.

Despite my attitude, the medical team continued to offer encouragement. After the hysterectomy, radiation might eradicate any remaining microscopic disease, they believed. They prescribed six weeks of radiation treatments in the abdominal area: five days a week, 90 seconds on one side, 90 seconds on the other, to begin in May.

Learning the details of radiation treatment felt like an interrogation session. The doctor sat on one side of a stark hospital room; I sat on the other, as though receiving sentence. He told me all the details of all the things that might go wrong, how sick I might be, how tough it would be. Then he let me go.

After those graphic descriptions, I called my surgeon.

"I can't have the radiation treatments. I don't have the strength to go through this," I said.

"Don't make up your mind immediately," he said. "I'll put you in touch with another doctor. Do some more thinking."

How could I decide which horror would be worse: the horror of side effects from radiation, or the horror of dying from a tumor I could have beaten? Since most of the cancer treatment is, ultimately, educated guesswork, cancer patients face these questions constantly. There is never a beam of light with the answer; ultimately, you are always very much alone when you make these decisions.

Working up a stoic courage, I agreed to radiation. When the radiation treatments started, I asked a hospital social worker where to find a support group for cancer patients.

"I don't know of one," she said, "but I'll look for one and get back to you."

She never did. And I didn't ask again.

That summer I walked past the fresh fruits and vegetables in the grocery stores, realizing in yet another way how much my life had changed. My friends, part of the natural-foods generation, were enjoying the summer's abundance. But the radiation so irritated my digestive system that fresh food was impossible.

Despite my emotional misery, exhausted and irradiated, I tolerated the six weeks of treatments "moderately well," the medical report said.

At the end of those five months, after the initial crisis of diagnosis, surgery, and radiation treatments, I felt 90 years old. I felt I would never regain energy, liveliness, perspective. I continued on stoically, trying to get on with my life. I stayed on my own that summer, living in that apartment and having to climb those stairs, feeling I had to keep my independence. How isolating, lonely, naive—sad—that I pushed away help. But I continued to deny the reality of the disease, hoping life would magically return to normal.

"I'll just overcome this," I told myself. "It will go away, and I can get on with my life, continue with things the way they used to be, without cancer."

"If I let go for one minute," I believed, "if I admit how frightened I am, I could collapse in a heap and never get up."

I determined to stay strong by sheer force of will: Get up in the morning, dress, go to work—even though I felt emotionally destroyed. I called it "coping."

This kind of denial—not openly grieving my loss, not accepting the care of family and friends—hurt me much more than I understood at the time. What I called "not dwelling on things" was actually a refusal to face a very difficult change in my life. My "coping" couldn't make the cancer go away, and I was allowing it to dominate my interior life.

Back on the job after radiation, I felt a growing dissatisfaction. I liked the college and my coworkers, but the work itself wasn't compelling. Being of service to others, a goal I had always admired, became an ideal I decided to actively pursue. I started social-work school, thinking an answer might lie there.

I began to think again about joining a cancer support group. My friends and family were there for me, of course, but I needed to talk with cancer patients, people who had been through cancer diagnosis, surgery, and radiation.

This time, a friend in the social-work program, recognizing my desperation, told me about Tom Welch, who led a support group for cancer patients. I was interested, but timid.

"I'll take you over there to meet people," she said.

The meetings changed my life. In October 1981, I joined the Focus Group and attended for more than three years. With friends there, I began to confront my fear of death, not by forcing death out of my consciousness, but by embracing, befriending, the fear and thus neutralizing its power. Those first 18 months of my illness, all that trying to run away, wasted so much energy that could have been used healing myself.

In the Focus Group, I learned that looking at my illness would not open a Pandora's box of woes that would swallow me whole. On the contrary, looking at the trauma in my life helped heal the wound. Not healing from the outside in, but healing from the inside out.

Emotionally, I had shut down, trying to avoid addressing the truth. Joining the Focus Group, I took my first small step up, out of the abyss.

During the first few months in the group, I listened to others, too shy to speak, wondering how to fit in. Supposedly, I was free of disease, recovered from the radiation treatments and recovered—physically at least—from the hysterectomy. Everyone else in the group struggled with active disease, and sometimes also with terminal diagnoses.

The awkward feeling, that perhaps I didn't need to be there, was compounded by my reaction to two other group members. John was nearing death from lung cancer. And an older woman, Beth, had had active breast cancer for more than a decade.

"Compared with John and Beth," I thought, "my problems are insignificant."

In fact, John and Beth presented my first pivotal lesson in living with cancer. Beth, bitter and angry, had cut herself off from friends, from work, and from most kinds of fun. She shut down, pulled down the shades, and sat at home, waiting to die.

"I've been living with cancer for more than 10 years, and

your diagnosis is new," she said to me. "You don't know yet what it's like."

Early on, I believed her. I listened, profoundly disturbed, convinced that, over the years, cancer would inevitably put an enormous strain on living and that fatigue and anger would dominate my life. She came on so strong that I believed joy, happiness, and fun would never again enter my life. Only anger and bitterness would remain.

Then John and I became friends. John, whom I knew for six months before he died, had been a teacher at a school for the blind. He used his last six months on earth to help me, to talk with his wife and family, to play with his son in the park, to keep in contact with close friends, and to be as alive and loving and vibrant as anyone I'd ever known.

John's approach to death was nonviolent. He talked about his sadness at not seeing his son grow up, about missing work and many things he had once planned on. But he spent his time living from day to day.

The day before his death, in the hospital, barely able to talk, John thought to ask how I was feeling. I told him what our friendship had meant to me; he listened and answered, despite his pain and fatigue. A special energy, an elusive but vital presence, came from him. He was more alive the day before his death than many people 20 years before their deaths.

John's death touched but did not devastate me. Physically, his time with me was very short, but his time with me spiritually has been very, very long. Through his peaceful approach to living with cancer and to dying, John taught an alternative to fighting for life out of anger—fighting for life out of a spiritual peacefulness. It seemed to me that John never needed to articulate his spirituality, but lived it instead. Others, recognizing the quality, were drawn to him. John's internal life spoke so much more loudly than any words or external actions.

After his death in May 1982, John left one more present— his own funeral. Everyone gathered at the Quaker meeting house, sitting on hard wooden benches facing each other. After a song of the Weston Priory monks, "All I ask of you is forever to remember me as loving you," friends stood to tell special stories about John. One woman remembered his shaving-cream habit: For many months, he bought the smallest can, expecting to die at any time.

"I knew something had changed inside him," the friend said, "when he started buying the large economy size."

John's gift of his own funeral showed friends and family that his love and sharing continued, even after his physical death. And so he showed us that feelings for people—thus the people themselves—do not die with the passing of the body.

From John and from Beth, I learned an essential primary lesson in living with cancer: There are many ways to face the challenge. People always have choices, even if the challenge is death. Beth talked in the Focus Group, filled with anger and bitterness, closed off from friends and family. Yet John, full of life as he grew closer to death, filled his life to overflowing with love and friendship. One saw the glass as half empty, the other as half full.

So I had a choice. I couldn't choose to live or die: We don't make that decision. But I could choose, as Elizabeth Kubler-Ross says, to live until I die.

I didn't suddenly reach this understanding and live happily ever after. I didn't receive a flash of enlightenment, find Nirvana, and feel fine forever after. I didn't even gradually grasp this concept of choice and come out from my hiding place to stay. Sometimes I just pulled up the covers. I still do from time to time. I have been scared, and I'm still scared.

But I did take the first tiny steps toward growth. I found a core group of cancer patients who became friends, friends with whom I could discuss my fears. People listened to my feelings, identified with them, and reciprocated.

The key here is "reciprocation." In America, we don't talk

publicly or easily about death, except to tell jokes. We are afraid of death. I could talk with Focus friends about death without burdening them, because they, too, faced that challenge.

The Focus Group taught many other lessons. For the first time, I told the whole story of my illness, from diagnosis to joining the group. In telling the story, completely and without interruption, I felt its full force consciously for the first time. Over time, voicing the feelings diminished their power over me.

The group helped in practical ways, also. Nurses and doctors often are too rushed to explain things in detail to each patient. Some patients may need or prefer information they can't find in books and those ubiquitous leaflets lying around doctors' offices. The Focus Group offered practical, on-the-job advice. More than a year later, I was still having intestinal problems, inconvenient and uncomfortable, from the radiation. I had endured them, coping with radiation side effects like the trouper I thought I was supposed to be, but people in the group gave me hints for getting along better.

The group helped also with the complexities of coping with medicine and doctors. I learned not to be satisfied with a medical professional who was patronizing, wouldn't return phone calls, or wouldn't answer questions. I learned to seek out opinions from other doctors. The group helped me assert myself, when necessary, with doctors, nurses, and other hospital staff. By networking, listening to stories and hearing how others handled their doctors, I learned what questions to ask, how to find information and how to refuse "No" or "I don't know" as answers.

"Don't give up," the Focus Group taught. It helped us realize that our questions, concerns, and fears were all valid, despite any negative reactions from medical staff. The more experienced cancer patients supported members newly diagnosed, frightened, and overwhelmed. From the veterans, new members learned to reject helplessness in favor of action:

Cancer patients can always choose options and take action, despite the illness.

In 1984 my cancer recurred. The medical team wanted to treat me with chemotherapy this time around. I wanted to know the names of the three drugs I would be taking. Unfortunately, I was having trouble communicating with my doctor, an excellent medical man. I initially had trouble getting him to answer telephone calls or to call me back. I kept calling and calling, wanting to know the names of the drugs so I could look them up.

"Call me back. Call me later," he kept saying.

One final time I got him on the phone.

"Call me back this afternoon at five," he said.

"No, that won't do," I said, surprising myself. "I was thinking more like noon."

There was a silence.

"OK," he said, "call me back at noon."

He explained the basic strategy of chemotherapy this way: "We want to give you enough chemo to kill off the cancer cells, but not enough to kill you. So there's a very fine line here."

Given a statement like that, I want to know as much as possible about what's going on, about what's being put into my body and about what's being done to my body. I trust my doctors, but in the end I must rely on my ability to take care of myself.

In that summer, 1984, I began five months of chemotherapy treatments. I hated them, but told myself I would withstand the treatments in order to control the tumor. With treatments once a month, I had one difficult week, followed by three that were slightly better.

After the third treatment, the medical team decided the tumor wasn't responding to the massive flood of toxic chemicals. Hearing that news, as I was preparing for the fourth treatment, I didn't have the energy to go through with something so difficult and seemingly so pointless. I went home that day to regroup, gather courage, and come back for another try the next day. At that point I felt, not hopeless, but discouraged, angry, and depressed. I had been a good patient, following orders and trying to help myself as much as possible.

The challenge of chemotherapy, the nausea and the fatigue of the cell-killing-off process, is so hard to meet. The chemo is designed to kill off a part of the person and, if we let it, it will kill off our spirit, too.

Once again, an obsession with death began sapping my vitality. If I wanted to follow John's example, I realized, if I wanted to remain alive until I died, I would have to stop this. I would have to get out of this limbo between death and life. I would have to take some action.

I did. I took a walk down Newbury Street.

Newbury Street, beginning at the edge of the Boston Public Garden, is an elegant avenue of shops, restaurants, and expensive boutiques. On sunny afternoons the street is crowded with people looking at store windows, restaurant menus, and each other.

One fine fall afternoon, I took off my wig and buckled a leather cat collar with rhinestones around my neck. I put pipe cleaners on my wrist for bracelets and put on the darkest eyeliner and mascara and the brightest makeup I could find.

My sister-in-law, dressed in a conservative pillbox hat, drove me and my young niece and nephew to Newbury Street and parked the car. We pretended I was the punked-out California baby-sitter and she was the quite conservative and very concerned New England mother, interviewing a prospective employee.

We got out of the car several blocks from the outdoor café where we planned to have ice cream in the warm fall sunlight. We started walking.

I had wanted to do something outrageous with my bald head. Where would a bald head look absolutely out of place? Newbury Street.

I never did like wearing a wig. The first time I wore mine, in the middle of a hot Boston summer, it felt like an elephant sitting on my head. I put it on to go to work and walked down Tremont Street with a friend to my office. I kept looking to see whether people were staring or not.

"There's no one even paying attention to my hair," I said finally.

"Of course not," she said. "You look fine."

I still hated the wig. It was summertime, hot and humid, and I couldn't wait every evening to get home, to put my thumb under the hairpiece and flip it off.

So why did I wear it? When I thought about it, I realized the strongest reason was that I didn't want people looking at me and feeling sorry for me. The Newbury Street caper was my own personal jailbreak, an escape from the constraints—physical, emotional, spiritual—of being considered a cancer "victim." This walk was designed to shout a message: The cancer and the chemo are not killing me off; maybe things have changed, but I can still have some fun.

So off we walked in the sunlight, my sister-in-law, my niece and nephew, five and six, and me, with my shiny bald head.

"Are you sure you'll be OK with the kids?" the anxious mother asked.

"Sure, sure. No problem, no problem . . . ," I kept saying, in a bored-teenager voice.

Going down the first block, one step in front of another, I kept my head down and played my role rather poorly, succumbing to opening-scene nervousness. I hardly dared look at anyone. Marching that second block, I started to relax and take a few cautious peeks at passersby. By the third block I was having a great time watching people's reactions. People were not looking at my hairless head and pitying me.

Instead, they thought I was just plain weird. When we walked into the café, the startled waiter nearly dropped his tray.

Business people on their lunch hour did double takes. Some of the older people looked downright angry at the tasteless younger generation. Foreign tourists took my picture: a typical Bostonian at an outdoor café.

Only the teenagers really got the joke. They stopped and laughed, realizing I was an adult caricature of their own culture, and tried to figure out if I was a clown or a nut. Instead of my bald head making people look away from me, pitying me and feeling ashamed of their own good health, the baldness drew people to me, either to glare at me or to smile indulgently.

This was fun. And I just had to get some fun out of the chemo. The limbo of existence, the discouragement from the chemo's failure, threatened to overwhelm me. Cancer might touch parts of my body, might even disfigure me, but my spirit could survive if I chose to let it.

Newbury Street was a statement: "Yes, I have cancer. But life does not stop at diagnosis and there will still be moments of pure joy."

I also got a great holiday card out of the afternoon. My sister-in-law took pictures at the café, featuring my cat collar and bald head. The café's white lights in the background resembled the delicate white lights of Christmas. I realized the snapshot would make a terrific holiday card, a nice memento of the experience. To me, the walk represented transcendence over the physical body, the essence of the spirit of Christmas.

Losing my hair wasn't the ultimate devastation to my body. The hair, at least, would grow back. Once I had that attitude, I played around with developing a flair for the dramatic. When it was growing back, about one-quarter inch long, I didn't wear scarves or a wig. One morning I was having breakfast in a Howard Johnson's.

"You are so brave to have your hair cut that short," a middle-aged woman said. "It looks wonderful."

"Where did you find someone in this country willing to

cut your hair that short? I had to go to Paris the last time I had
my hair cut like that," a woman in a health club said.

At the end of the chemo treatments, my friend Joan
celebrated with a gathering in my honor. Actually, it was a
network meeting, a gathering of the tribe. She called together
some friends, to spend an evening at my house, singing, talking,
and eating. And to talk about the next step, after the failed
chemo.

"In a primitive culture," Joan began, "when a member is
in trouble, the tribe comes together. Lisa has a challenge ahead
of her. The energy of the whole is more than the sum of its parts.
Together, therefore, as a group, we can give her something she
may not be able to find on her own."

"I create black-and-white thinking," I told the group,
speaking tentatively at first. "I make up things like: 'I'm never
going to get any better.' I need my friends to remind me that I
won't always feel this way, that someday I can feel happy again
and have courage. I need my friends to remind me that my
discouragement is temporary."

Perhaps, I told my friends, some friends may not want to
know me. They may be frightened by this recurrence in my
illness.

"I need assurances that you won't disappear now," I told
them, speaking painfully about very private terrors.

Then I began speaking about the worst fear of all—death.

"Being alone at night is so hard right now," I said. "When
things get very frightening, when I can't control my thoughts, I
have no one to talk to."

Someone offered to be available for phone conversation
at three or four in the morning, so I could call when the
heebie-jeebies hit. Others offered to do other things, like cook.

"These people are committed to me," I thought. "They
aren't saying yes to something I've asked for; they are saying yes
before I have a chance to ask."

That made all the difference in the world. Asking for

extras, when you are ill, is so hard. You already feel like such
a burden to others. When my friends made the first move,
initiating the meeting and asking to be part of my life, I felt
differently. I learned I was giving them a gift, by allowing them
to be with me during this difficult time. All these people—my
friends—brought together fabulous resources and talents and
were waiting to be allowed to use them.

The network gathering energized my friends, too, because they met a group of people committed to my welfare.
Individually, they might have felt frustrated about giving me
enough time and attention. But as a group, they felt empowered
to accomplish a common goal.

After the walk down Newbury Street and the networking
party, I reenergized and adopted some new strategies: attending cancer-related workshops and college courses, and seeking
out more information on concepts of holistic health. Several
friends had encouraged me to attend these workshops, but I
had resisted, feeling they were too simplistic. Guilt-inducing,
even, since I interpreted the idea of being "responsible" for my
illness as my having caused the cancer and being at fault for it.
But with the failure of the chemo, I needed help.

I agreed to go to a weekend workshop led by Bernie
Siegel, who kept talking about hugging your doctor. It's important, he said, to make a connection, an emotional connection, with the doctor that goes beyond treating disease.

I didn't know I was going to do it. After an exam, on the
spur of the moment, heading out the door, I turned around.

"Would you mind giving me a hug?" I said to my doctor.

"No," he answered, and gave me a hug. He didn't seem
surprised, and didn't misunderstand what I was asking for.

Years later, it's still part of our routine.

"Don't forget the hug. It's important," he says to me
before I leave his office.

After the hug, my doctor started sharing more things. Now
he tells me if he's had a lousy day, instead of letting me figure

it out for myself. Once he said he thought I was in better shape than he was. We see through the roles, to our mutual humanity. I know he cares about me, and he knows I care about him.

Dealing with life and death issues, I needed more from him than drugs. I needed to feel he cared whether I lived or died. Sometimes, doctors look at disease and, perhaps, miss the whole person. Patients look at the doctor as God, missing the natural, human limitations. With neither communicating at a human level, a valuable part of the relationship vanishes. The doctor needs to feel that the patient cares and isn't always going to be demanding things that a doctor may be limited in giving— more time, a complete cure.

Another workshop I attended was a weekend retreat, recommended by Joan, called "Opening the Heart." I went pretty soon after the chemo treatments, when I was run down, tired, bald, and emotionally worn out.

"I'd really like it if you took your scarf off," someone told me the second day. "It seems like you're hiding something."

The covering came off, to reveal my bald head. The unspeakable was made bare. This was very different from Newbury Street, where I retained anonymity despite my exhibitionism. This was within a small group of people who knew my name and who knew my story.

Oddly enough, after uncovering on that personal and intimate level, I felt more open, more at ease. If others could accept the shocking effects of my illness, surely I could also. By removing the scarf, I uncovered myself externally to parallel an internal uncovering, as I began to integrate my interior and exterior selves.

The weekend brought about a healing, not a physical healing from cancer but an emotional and psychological healing.

During this whole period, my doctors were debating the next step in treatment. They discussed intraperitoneal chemotherapy—"bellybath" chemo—and another option with a 25 percent mortality rate.

"No thanks," I said.

Surgery was discussed, but my original surgeon wanted to hold off on another major surgical procedure as long as possible. "Wait and watch," seemed to be the general consensus. So for about a year I had this tumor growing inside me, difficult to remove surgically and impossible to affect with chemotherapy.

I knew it was there, going untreated. The idea of death obsessed me. Its power over me occupied far too much of my time. To be released, I knew, I would have to face death, confront it, almost befriend it. This was possible, I knew. John had given me the gift of his knowledge.

Trying to overcome my obsession, I took a college course, "Opening to Death," with a friend who also had cancer. The other students in the course were future counselors or clergy, people who might work with dying patients. My friend and I brought an emotion-filled, real-life atmosphere to the class.

Thinking about my own possibly imminent death was very painful. I cried through the first section of one meditation, but gradually the warmth and light of meditation absorbed my attention, and I felt an unlimited horizon of heart space. It was very comforting to feel that limitless space, unbounded by the mind, and I stopped crying. For the first time, I understood a kind of essential truth: I had been bounded throughout my physical life by limiting walls and barriers. Walls of imagination and barriers of the mind. During this meditation, the limits began dropping away. The unbounded feeling, the openness I felt fleetingly during that meditation, was a comfort.

This sense of the disintegration of physical limitations was a key experience in shaping my future, an experience which would return in future crises. Life, I learned, is something different from my usual, everyday, three-dimensional perception. The essence of life is not the human body, but an integration of body, mind, and spirit.

In February 1986, the tumor began obstructing my intestines. My medical team prescribed more radiation, so I climbed up on the radiation table to have my body tattooed for treatment. While I was on the table—after my body was permanently tattooed—the radiologists discovered from an x-ray that my bowel lay directly in the radiation field. The team didn't want to risk inflicting further radiation on the delicate intestinal tissues. Radiation was out as a treatment option. I was furious at the permanent and now useless tattooing of my body.

So I returned to my initial surgeon.

"Surgery would be a major undertaking," he said. "I don't advise it until absolutely necessary."

But you reach a point of intolerance when you cannot bear the cancerous tissue growing unchecked inside you. I had reached that point.

"Why wait until you're in an emergency and not physically strong enough to deal with surgery?" my oncologist said.

To get other opinions outside the Boston medical establishment, I decided to go to Sloan-Kettering Memorial Cancer Center in New York City. This wasn't because I didn't trust my Boston medical team. But getting opinions from people at different hospitals, in different cities even, can provide a more complete picture.

One doctor at Sloan-Kettering I will never forget. After discussing my case with his assistant, I entered his office, pulled out my list of questions, and began.

"It's too bad," the doctor said. "It's too bad you're doing it the way you're doing it."

"What do you mean?" I asked, thinking he might have some helpful suggestion.

"It's too bad you don't just sit back and be the patient and let us handle things."

I was absolutely furious. Traveling to New York for treatments would have been difficult, but I would have done it. I knew, though, that I could never work with someone with such an attitude. After all the gains I'd made, I wasn't about to sit back and be passive.

It's not just some doctors who have that condescending attitude. One Boston nurse consistently spoke that way. I was used to tracking results of the CA125 blood test, which researchers believe indicates the level of active ovarian cancer cells in the body. After one blood test, the nurse refused to tell me the CA125 level.

"You don't need to know those numbers," she said. "They're for the doctor, not you."

She told me they were "normal."

"What does 'normal' mean?" I asked. "What are the numbers?"

"You won't understand them if I tell you," she insisted. "They have to be taken in context with other medical information."

I want to participate in the whole process of living with cancer, including understanding tests. I need to track the information, to better understand medical decisions. It is my own body. I need to know what the thinking is, because ultimately I make the decision—not the doctor. I sign the consent form, and I suffer the consequences of the side effects. (After a lengthy conversation, the nurse agreed to send the test results.)

Another Sloan-Kettering doctor suggested hormonal therapy, which my Boston oncologist agreed to try. The hormones worked. The tumor shrank. For almost a year, the tumor continued to shrink. Six months into treatment, part of the weakened tumor, breaking down, became cystic. In July 1987, surgeons operated, hoping to remove the remains of the tumor.

Instead, they found more disease than expected, requiring more extensive surgery, including the removal of some colon. A colostomy could result. Rather than perform the surgery without psychologically preparing me, my surgeon closed the 12-inch incision without removing anything. Further surgery was scheduled for September.

Ten days later, while I was recuperating at home, a friend telephoned.

"A Filipino psychic surgeon is in Washington," she said. "You should try to go immediately, fly down."

"I have trouble and pain even moving around the house," I said. "How can I go to Washington or get on a plane?"

But, driven by hope, I did go. Another friend with cancer traveled with me. At the airport I had to have a wheelchair. Despite my exhaustion, we went straight to the Filipino healer.

About 25 people were waiting to see him, checked in by a woman claiming to have been cured of terminal lung cancer. Services were free, but donations were accepted.

In the examining room, with his wife and niece as assistants, the man said he would open my belly using psychic techniques and take out damaged tissue. He used no instruments, relying only on his hands. I felt no pain, but some pressure. I went several times during the next two days. In one session there was considerable pressure, as though he were really digging down. Afterward, I felt quite weak and exhausted.

"What about the surgery in September?" I asked the Filipino the last time I saw him. "Should I do it?"

"You will know in September what to do," he answered. "I will pray for you."

I left him filled with a sense of confidence that I could indeed trust my own intuition, trust my own heart. The visit renewed my hope—hope that I could trust myself to know what to do. This hope was not for a miracle cure, not for reassurance that "it'll be all right." The hope I regained was that, whatever happened in the coming months, I would be able to cope. I would be able to continue my emotional and spiritual life, despite the coming physical hardships.

Someone who offers hope offers something very real and very essential to the healing process. But it's up to us cancer patients to know what we're hoping for. I didn't hope this man would cure me, but I did hope something would shift in me in some way: spiritual, emotional, physical.

I don't know if he actually reached inside my body. He did a demonstration for us that looked as though he did. However, I've also heard of a magician doing that same demonstration, explaining it as illusion. No matter. The mechanics are less important than the healing that, unquestionably, occurred within me. After the July surgery I was very, very low. I was facing extensive cancer, more mutilating surgery, great physical losses.

After the psychic surgery I felt much better, emotionally and spiritually. I came down to Washington in a wheelchair. Three days later I was running—albeit at a 45 degree angle—to catch a plane. The spiritual work diverted my focus from physical pain and discomfort, helping me overcome the limits of the physical body.

This would happen again for me, very soon, in an even more powerful way, during an even more serious physical crisis. In September, my surgeon removed the tumor in the colon. In October, I was hospitalized because of a fistula (perforation) in the intestinal wall, probably weakened as a result of tumor growth, surgery, and radiation. Despite a liquid diet, prescribed to ease the fistula's healing, my body could not absorb nutrients. I was suffering from malnutrition.

Hospitalization was Thursday. Friday I received a mainline catheter for intravenous feeding. Monday I received a colostomy. Several days later, my arms and neck swelled from a blood clot. A shortage of oxygen, probably caused by fluid in my lungs and medication, brought on mental confusion. One night I kept trying to climb out of bed and escape the hospital, saying I was being held hostage.

The list kept growing. Aside from the basic cancer, I had suffered from a recto-vaginal fistula, from malnutrition, from a blood clot in my left arm, from a confused state, from fluid in the lungs, from an infection that escaped from the bladder, through the kidneys and into the bloodstream.

Next, a radiologist said I might have a fistula in the bladder. An aide left me alone on a gurney in the hospital hall to absorb that news.

"I'm weak and growing weaker." Overwhelmed, I began fantasizing. "All my tissues are falling apart. Eventually I will just disintegrate. Can I tolerate life like this?" I asked myself desperately.

Fifteen minutes later, Jim Grant walked in. I had known Jim for several years, since he had seen the Christmas card of my Newbury Street escapade at a friend's house. Working over the years with Jim, a spiritual teacher, I began understanding that I was a spiritual being. And I began learning how to tap into the essence of that spiritual energy—my higher power.

In the hospital room, Jim listened as I told him about the physical crises of the past several days. Then he shifted planes. He was still listening, but he was listening from a different place. Not consciously aware, I mirrored his focus.

The walls, the boundaries of physical life, fell away. I found a place not affected by the physical and emotional, a place with a limitless horizon.

"Yes," I found myself thinking, "my body might die. But here's this limitless possibility for the spirit. This is a new kind of strength, a place of peacefulness, joy, and serenity."

This sense of limitless spirit renewed my energy and hope. The hope lay not in my body getting better, but in my new understanding that whatever happened, I would find the strength to move ahead with life. This place of spiritual strength helps me know that I will go on with life. The essence of me is neither my body nor my mind, but my spirit.

Before cancer, I felt I would fall apart at the slightest challenge. In the early years of cancer, with the help of a very caring therapist and my support group, I learned about emotional strength. Now I am learning about spiritual strength, and even enjoying new challenges in living.

My overall perspective has widened into realms beyond the day-to-day, beyond the physical. When the pain and fear return, now I know I can access that special space. I know I can cope with the challenges of body and mind, and I carry the feelings that were generated by the meditation on my own death, by the visit to the psychic surgeon, by the focusing experience with Jim.

I don't know if my spiritual development has affected the cancer. Ultimately, we may not know these things. But I know that my growing understanding of spirit has affected my general health. In the hospital, focusing on a higher power with Jim, I became much less anxious, much less emotionally debilitated, more able to roll with the punches.

Despite ovarian cancer, I have many choices in life; I am only as trapped as I allow myself to be. I have many medical resources, a variety of social and emotional choices, and an ever-present spiritual path that I am only now beginning to know.

Suicide, when I was first diagnosed, seemed the only alternative I had to a life doomed to misery and pain. The thought still crosses my mind. But not so often. I possess a different kind of knowledge now. I know now that dying will be a process for which I feel more prepared.

It's very rewarding to come through the dark times. After all the pain and fear and horrible fantasies, to be sitting here in this moment is well worth the struggle. Tiny step by tiny step, it all seems worthwhile.

EPILOGUE

As of October 1989, Lisa had no discernible trace of cancer. Her oncologist, Steven Come, Director of Oncology

Units at Boston's Beth Israel Hospital and faculty member at Harvard Medical School, talked about the case.

"It's difficult to say what will happen with Lisa's tumor, a low-grade tumor with a slow course. The survival rate for these tumors at 10 years is about 5 to 7 percent," Come said.

Lisa had some difficult complications with the surgery that removed several nodules of recurrent cancer in the septum between the rectum and the vagina, he added.

"We wanted to do the surgery while the cancer was still potentially operable," Come said. "To date, there's been no evidence of recurrence. But we're not out of the woods yet."

Lisa has remained a vital participant in her own treatment, despite those difficulties, he continued.

"Initially, Lisa had some problem with depression. This has been a test for her, and she has become a rock," he said. "At some point, she decided she wasn't going to throw in the towel. She's either going to contribute to making herself better or go down fighting. Since then, she has taken a lot of responsibility for her own health, which I encourage.

"I'm not sure it makes the cancer better. But even if it doesn't kill a single cancer cell, it certainly helps the patient tolerate it."

Come said he has not discouraged Lisa's investigation of other avenues of healing aside from those he has prescribed.

"I have to be skeptical that attitudes can get rid of cancer," he said. "But, along with bovine liver extract and the rest of that stuff, she's never refused to do anything I've asked her to do.

"Do I think these remedies are useful, based on what I learned at Harvard Medical School? No. But am I sure they won't help? No. I do know that peace of mind is important. And I like the idea of her being interested in her care. Far from resenting her interest as an intrusion, I wish more people were like that. If I were in her shoes, I hope I'd act that way too."

Lisa's surgeon, Arlan Fuller, on the faculty of Harvard Medical School and on the staff of Massachusetts General Hospital, said Lisa has been especially successful in living with cancer.

"Despite the seriousness of her illness, Lisa has been tremendously successful—successful in terms of her ability to live a worthwhile life and in terms of what she has done for other patients," Fuller said.

In the spring of 1989, Lisa celebrated her fortieth birthday by walking 10 miles in Boston's annual Walk for Hunger, a subscription walk to raise money for local food programs.

Julie Cavadini

INTRODUCTION

At 29, with only two weeks to live according to one doctor's prediction, Julie Cavadini picked up two plain sheets of white paper. On one, she wrote "reasons to live"; on the other, "reasons to die."

"Reasons to live" finally contained more lines than "reasons to die." Not many more, but enough to tip the balance.

At 31, Julie tells her story. Tyler, Julie's husband and an intrinsic part of her decision to live, also participates in this narrative.

Julie's Story

Julie

Don't confuse surrender with capitulation. Surrendering to the power of death is a necessary part of living. Not until you accept death—join life and death into a unity—do you begin to get well.

Walking along the beach last fall, I found a seagull dying. The bird lay on its side, scratching its beak frantically in the gritty sand. Lifting its head from side to side, the gull pecked the air fearfully, craving escape.

Terrified and hypnotized, I watched, wondering what to do. Saving the bird, defending life and cheating death, seemed essential. Then I realized I was there to observe, not act. Sitting far enough from the bird to keep from disturbing it, I expected a long wait. Death must take time. It must be an immense and monumental process, requiring many hours.

The bird circled its long neck round and round several times, hid its head under a wing, drew three long breaths—and died. Death was so startlingly simple, the surrendering a natural culmination to life. Surrender like that, appropriate and timely, is not capitulation. It's an acceptance, an allowance. The gull's final peace made a powerful statement.

Burying the bird, I remembered my own fight for life, my own refusal to capitulate—and my own surrender. Now, at 31, I have learned self-trust.

Tyler and I married in the fall of 1984, just a few days before my 28th birthday. Tyler managed a bike shop and played guitar; I taught piano and composition at a state college. During several years of living together, we talked, infrequently, about marriage; I preferred the status quo. Taking risks or making commitments weren't high on my agenda; marriage looked like an ending of freedom, rather than a beginning.

That summer my father began treatments for cancer, lymphoma, and I decided to make the commitment to Tyler. We set a wedding date for that fall.

Tyler loved me—that's the way he is—but I still had many doubts about this wedding. We planned a small and simple wedding, with an even smaller reception. Some of my friends and family are still upset, but we had no room to invite everyone.

"This is the worst thing I've ever done in my life. Why am I doing this?" I kept thinking during the two months of planning.

The emotions of the wedding ceremony were unexpected and strong. Tyler's father, ordained a Baptist minister, performed the ceremony in a Catholic church with a priest beside him, to honor my Catholic family. He talked for a very long time about our marriage, about our feelings for each other.

In a church you're supposed to feel the presence of God. That day, listening to Tyler's father, I felt that presence for the first time. It was so strong, so unexpected, so obvious.

"Something very sacred is happening here," I kept thinking during the ceremony. "It feels like this union is truly blessed. Just like they say."

Six months later, doctors said I was dying from leukemia.

Tyler

I came home from a day-long bike trip with a buddy. Julie was in pain. She was doubled over, having trouble breathing. I took her to the local emergency room, where the doctor felt her side and did some tests.

"Your wife is very sick," he said, taking me aside.

"What do you mean?" I said. "She hasn't been sick."

"Your wife has leukemia," he said.

Time stopped.

Julie

The doctor gave Tyler the privilege of announcing the diagnosis, which is what he would have preferred anyway. Tyler looked so scared.

"Don't worry," I told him. "They're wrong."

The emergency room doctor looked pretty upset too.

"Don't worry. It isn't so bad," I joked with him, and then asked about taking a birth control pill the next morning. He stared, unblinking, like the question was incredible.

"She doesn't get this," he was thinking. "She just doesn't get it."

Actually, I just didn't believe them. People in their 20s don't get leukemia. There had been no prior illness, besides recent headaches and fatigue coming from too much teaching. Anyway, newlyweds don't get fatal illnesses.

From the small local hospital, I went to spend seven days in a New Haven hospital room, with a roommate who also had cancer. Hospitals are definitely not places to get well. All night long the man across the hall screamed in pain. All day long people came in and out of the room to prick, poke, and prod for any number of unexplained reasons.

Those seven depressing days in that hospital wore me down. I had to believe the doctors. I had leukemia.

Leukemia is cancer of the blood-forming organs, the lymph glands and the bone marrow. It's an unbalancing of the body: Too many white cells are made, pushing out the red cells. My leukemia is chronic myelitic leukemia, supposed to proceed in three phases, from chronic to accelerated to blast. It's an adult leukemia, different from what the kids get, and takes many years to develop.

By the time the disease is obvious, the out-of-control cell division has progressed pretty far, pushing out most of the normal cells.

That summer, the doctors believed I had nearly completed the chronic phase, after a development of about nine years. They estimated the accelerated phase, one generally much shorter and more severe, would begin soon. Acceleration, the doctors said, is fatal.

Tyler

After they took Julie to New Haven, I finally got to sleep at six in the morning. I slept only a few hours and woke up thinking. All I could think about was contacting someone who works with visualization. Julie and I had been interested in physical fitness, good nutrition, and mind-body health for a long while, although we never dreamed how important it was to become to us. I didn't know much about visualization, or anything about cancer at all, for that matter. But visualization seemed like a good way to begin to gather our spiritual strength.

I knew there was someone around who worked with visualization. I asked a doctor, who gave the impression he knew, but he didn't approve and wouldn't tell me.

One of the nurses walking by overheard the conversation.

"Oh," she said, when the doctor had left. "You mean Bernie, Bernie Siegel."

She handed me a telephone number.

Julie

Bernie came by, and he was just glowing. Doctors coming into hospital rooms generally bring bad news. They want something—blood or a test or to give unwelcome news. Patients develop Pavlovian responses of queasy stomachs to having doctors in their hospital rooms.

Bernie came in just to talk. He asked how I felt, and I said "Fine," not knowing then to tell the truth: "Lousy." I was trying so hard to be a good patient. Bernie gave me visualization and relaxation tapes, and his assistant, also named Julie, visited several times.

Tyler

From the beginning, my wife had an ability to affect her illness that surprised the doctors. After six days in the hospital, Julie asked her oncologist when she could go home. She hated that hospital and wanted out.

"You have a fever," he told Julie. "You have to be fever free for 24 hours before you can go home."

An hour later the fever was gone. Julie came home the next day. That was May 1985, and Julie hasn't been overnight in a hospital since then. We both hate hospitals and want her at home, where she won't have exotic drugs and she can be in peace.

Julie

Hospitals are like jails. You can't just walk out without your doctor signing you out, or the insurance company won't pay your bill. They really have you there. The idea is to stay out in the first place.

After the hospital, there were several visits with a woman connected to the cancer support group. She recommended joining the group, an idea I resisted because I was uncomfortable in groups of strangers. But I knew illness comes as a teacher, as a medium for change and growth. Living in a hospital is somewhat like living in a foreign country, or living in a war zone. It's a whole new world, with new rules and new cues, stunning in its isolation from the familiar world.

To survive the shock I had to change, to take risks and begin depending on people. The first steps were faltering, tiny but necessary. During those first six or seven weeks of group sessions, I said nothing but listened to everyone. Several women there had lived through near-death experiences. They talked so calmly about the ebbs and flows of life, about the reality of dying. They even made jokes about death, laughing about giving things away.

I had never been in any kind of group before, not even Girl Scouts. Speaking to people, having them all listen to me, let alone laughing about my own illness and death, seemed beyond my powers.

"You're very quiet," Bernie said one day. "How can we help you if you don't say anything?"

So I told them the previous night's dream. I'm always having dreams, many of them very strange, and Tyler and I talk about them the next morning, deciding what they mean. In this dream, Tyler and I lived in my grandfather's house, with the garden, as always, growing out back. But instead of carrots, I had planted several rows of penises.

The dream was about seeking the root of life, trying to understand disease and life and growth, Tyler and I had decided that morning at breakfast. Having never said a word, I was suddenly telling these people this outrageous dream.

Everyone laughed hysterically, but they were also surprised and quite shocked. I had looked, before I started talking, like such a nice, sweet girl.

Making a group of people laugh about cancer and my illness was taking a giant step toward confidence in myself and toward being part of the group. After that I talked frequently. And I had so much to learn. The others, in different stages of their journeys, had so much to teach. When they spoke about contradicting a doctor's orders, it was my turn to be shocked. Disagreeing with a doctor then seemed so radical to me, although it's just basic assertiveness. Learning to be angry about being sick, learning to be assertive, learning to fight for life, required at least a year of work with the group.

Anger and fear were negative emotions, I believed, and depression in the face of illness was a sign of weakness. Those negative emotions were feelings best kept to myself and better not to have at all. Independence, courage, and outward strength were what I thought I needed.

Cancer changed all that. I became a needy person, a person who needed others and who had to learn to love to survive.

"If you had only a year to live, what would you do?" Bernie kept asking.

I resented that question. It was too close, too raw. I wasn't willing to talk about that.

"What would make it so that, when you wake up in the morning, you look at your whole day with joy?" he asked.

I couldn't answer that. I was so other-oriented, set on achieving in my music career. I taught 50 hours a week, practiced, gave classes. I was a Wonder Woman: "I can do all this, and have cancer, too." I even spent one day a week working in a tiny office as a receptionist. Everyone smoked, so there I was, fighting cancer, wishing I could be a composer, and breathing in cigarette smoke all day long.

No wonder he wouldn't give up with the questions. I was just not willing to look at what I was doing, not willing to take chances trusting my own inner wisdom.

In October 1985, six months after diagnosis, my oncologist suggested a consultation at a cancer research center in Boston to consider a bone marrow transplant.

The body's white blood cells come from originating stem cells in the bone marrow. To do a transplant, massive doses of radiation first destroy—kill—all the stem cells, the healthy as well as the cancerous. Then, doctors inject donor cells into the bloodstream, hoping they will settle in the bone marrow and thrive. The healthy donor cells assume the job of the cancerous, now eradicated cells, if all goes well.

Several complications accompany this procedure. First, a donor with a very close tissue match must be willing to volunteer cells. Second, during the period between the killing of the original white cells and the healthy thriving of the donor cells, the body is very, very susceptible to disease, without protective immune system white cells on patrol. Third, the implanted cells could attack the body, in a serious and often fatal "graft-versus-host" reaction.

Finally, if all goes well, you must take immunosuppressent drugs for the rest of your life to keep the two cell types from attacking each other.

Even the American Cancer Society calls this extremely new treatment "drastic." The Society's *Cancer Book*, published at about the same time I considered the treatment, says "Transplants are now reserved for patients with disease that is resistant to standard therapy. They are performed at only four or five institutions across the United States, and have in some instances reversed an otherwise hopeless situation."

So the book is saying, first, that standard therapy wouldn't do me any good and, second, that I ranked among those patients in an "otherwise hopeless situation." That's what the Boston transplantation doctor was saying, too. I asked about waiting a year, until January 1987.

"I don't advise that," he said. "We'd lose you that way."

He wasn't betting on even one year. That's what this man was saying. I read everything available on the procedure, which wasn't much since it was so new. There weren't that many long-term survivors, which limited information on the quality of life after. The transplant itself carried a 30 to 40 percent mortality rate, not the greatest odds.

When I asked about having children, they said I would be sterile. Anyway, they added, they wouldn't advise it because of the life-expectancy of the mother. Again, people offered subtle predictions of death from this illness, one way or another.

The ticket just looked too expensive to take the ride.

Tyler

It seemed barbaric. They wouldn't even talk about the quality of life after it all. She was a prime candidate, unusually young and healthy aside from the cancer. This man was looking not at my Julie, but at a prime research candidate. Julie had to make her own decision. But if she had only a year to live, I hoped she'd have that year with only one or two physical problems, not completely debilitated.

Julie

It turned out that my brother was a perfect tissue match. This wasn't necessarily good news, because it meant the decision lay totally with me. It also meant the Boston doctors were more enthusiastic than ever: A young, otherwise healthy research candidate with a perfect tissue match—hopelessly ill enough to justify experimentation—is a rarity.

This was a horrible decision to have to make, terrible. The whole thing is framed in terms of death, not life. The doctor can't make the decision. And God doesn't come down and say: "Do this!" My family couldn't make the decision, which was difficult for my brother, who wanted to donate the cells as his way of helping.

The cancer group discussed the transplant endlessly.

"If you know you're going to die," someone asked, "why wouldn't you try the transplant?"

The issue crystallized. I didn't know I was going to die. That was the doctor's agenda, not mine. I had no intention of dying, of capitulating early without an argument. And I had better things to do than lie around dying from major experimental surgery.

The issue focused on: Trust me, or trust them. Even if my life would be shorter, the quality would be better, living by my own feelings. This transplant sounded exotic, full of incredible technology, depressing statistics, and endless and complicated medication regimes.

I knew, through being in group, self-trust and risk taking were essential. But this was the first time I ever had to take a risk on which my life was based. The cancer and the transplant question forced me to find my own convictions and follow my own truths.

On December 12, 1985, I refused the transplant. The decision was right—not because it kept me alive longer but because it kept me true to my own convictions. Trusting those feelings gave me confidence and energy. I give less attention to fear now, because I've been through the fire.

After that decision, the focus changed. I no longer concentrated on living longer: I concentrated on loving while I lived. I dreamt I was a big oak tree, so leafy and healthy that even if I lost a limb, I would be fine.

During this time of developing self-confidence and inner wisdom, I had to fight the negative opinions of others. My family respected my decision, but others tried to change my mind. Even my car mechanic told me to have the transplant.

"Why haven't you had the transplant yet?" a nurse at the hospital asked once while I was receiving a transfusion. "You know it's your only hope."

Hope lies inside your own soul: No one else can take your hope away. But when the nurse said that, I fell into a very severe depression, couldn't eat, wouldn't talk to anyone, didn't look at all the beautiful flowers friends sent.

A piano student, a little girl, arrived for a lesson on her birthday.

"I'm 10," she said. "I'm in the double digits now. I guess I'll be there the rest of my life."

"Unless you live to be 100," I said.

"No. I can't do that. I'll die before that."

"Why can't you?" I pushed. "What do people die from?"

"Cancer," she answered.

There it was again, all around me, that ubiquitous sense of general hopelessness connected with cancer. Learning to be true to my own confidence, despite others, became a full-time occupation. Everyone faces death. Feeling like a cancer "victim" only limited the joy and energy of my living.

That winter, February 1986, my father and I went to a hockey game for the evening. Riding up the escalator, I leaned over the side to watch some people on the down escalator. Suddenly a stranger grabbed me and threw me to the other side of the stairs. I had narrowly missed colliding with the wall where the up and down staircases crossed.

"A simple occurrence like that could wipe me out, after all this worry," I thought. "I'm really not any worse off than anyone else. What's the point of self-pity?"

That whole year I continued to teach, to practice, to work one day a week in that smoky office, and to attend group. Although jazz composition remained the ultimate achievement in my mind, I wasn't willing to make time to do it. Engrossed in the exterior life of career, achievement, and earning money, I was still in the "Wonder Woman" phase: "All this—and cancer, too."

In July 1986, the doctors said I had two weeks to live. That's when I surrendered to death—accepted death—and began to get well.

I was seeing a homeopathic doctor then, refusing chemotherapy, working too hard, not taking care of myself. I was feeling tired and run down, dangerously so. But I let the situation go for too long, probably because of an unwillingness to face up to things.

I kept hearing those "year-at-the-most," "hopeless case" predictions. According to those guys, my time was just about through. With predictions like that, what's the point of fighting?

Alarmed by my growing fatigue and worsening attitude, my homeopathic doctor ordered a blood test. The pathologist phoned immediately.

"You have a dying patient on your hands," he said. The count was up to 310,000.

After a second aspiration, the oncologist determined that the disease had moved into the accelerated phase. Two weeks, he said, not directly but subtly.

"I just can't do this anymore," I said to myself. I was so sick, so tired. I accepted death.

Tyler

Julie wanted to stay out of the hospital. I nursed her at home. We wanted her to have her own peace of mind, to not have to take extreme drugs or listen to the lonely noise of a hospital floor.

For days she lay on the couch, not moving, not really

present. I took her temperature every 15 minutes, bathed her, fed her. The homeopathic doctor came for an hour every evening, just to be there. The family came by often.

She developed an incredible fever, 105.6. She started sitting up, talking away with so much energy, so lucidly. I packed her in wet cloths, tried to cool her down in the tub. All the time, she was talking away like she was fine.

I asked her then if she was ready to say good-bye. I felt it was necessary to give her that freedom, that she wouldn't be worrying about me. If she needed to die, I wanted to let her.

The fever dropped. Then broke. Then the blood count dropped.

Julie

I was getting better. Before the fever, I had made up these lists: "reasons to live," "reasons to die."

The "live" list was longer than the "die" list. Not by much, but the difference was enough. I wanted to live to learn more about loving. I had never been absolutely sure about loving Tyler before. When I became sure, I didn't want to give that up.

And I didn't want to give up on loving myself. There were some workshops I wanted to attend that fall, some important things I needed to learn. I didn't choose to accept their predictions of death. I decided the doctors' agenda didn't have to be mine.

When I went to my oncologist's office for my next visit, he was astounded and delighted.

In August, on a week's vacation in Maine, I began to feel on the upswing. Natural surroundings can accomplish that. Tyler worried about going, because we had just heard this two-week thing less than a month ago. He worried about having to make a mad dash back home in an emergency. But I knew I was getting better.

That fall I attended the workshops I had promised myself.

Earlier in the illness, I had visited a reader, who had said I would get well and that I would learn a lot in the process. I met Flo, the reader, shortly after my diagnosis. While the doctors were talking about fatal illness, she talked about learning and growth. She helped me find something to believe in, something to look forward to.

That fall in Flo's workshop, I learned how to make noise. During that week-long workshop, I screamed. Before, to cry, I would go into my room and cry quietly, so no one would know. At the workshop, everyone made a circle. You had to get into the middle of the circle and do something. I was terrified, but I knew I had to do it. I went into the circle—and screamed for 90 minutes.

I was beginning to learn to be angry about the illness, learning to love and take risks. I was learning to be a real person. I think one reason I didn't die during that period is that I was having too much fun.

Tyler

That Christmas, 1986, I came back from a business trip and found Julie just glowing.

I hadn't seen her so happy in a long, long time. She had found a seven-foot Steinway grand piano that she thought she could buy. Christmas is Julie's favorite time of year and this piano had been finished on Christmas Eve, 1885. We decided to borrow the money and to make room in the house for it.

Julie

Christmas that year was wonderful. It was filled with all the excitement and fun of a kid's Christmas. I love buying presents and decorating trees. It's hectic but I just love it.

After Christmas I had another blood test. The count was

normal, a completely normal count with no abnormalities, the first normal count since the illness began.

The count was an enigma to the doctors. But I know why it was normal. Christmas is my favorite time of year. I was relaxed, not teaching during the holidays, and I thought I would be able to have that piano. My whole life was joyful.

Then I returned to teaching and work. The woman who owned the piano decided against selling it. I taught 35 students each week. I thought that since I was starting my career, I shouldn't refuse any requests. I was still doing that once-a-week office job. The blood count went up again.

And again, that next summer, I was seriously ill. But this time the doctors made no predictions.

"You've already outlived the statistics," the oncologist said. "I don't know what's going on with you. I'm not saying anything."

During this past year, the blood count has gone up and down. I'm not really attached to those numbers anymore, since I know they don't mean much. My own healing, the healing of my soul, is going well. I know that.

I took a semester off from teaching during the fall of 1987. For three months I spent time with just myself. My mother made dinner, arriving every night at about 5:30. That was the only thing scheduled. I was in such hibernation that I wouldn't even answer the phone. I was so protective of my space that Tyler and I slept in separate rooms. It was all a part of unwrapping myself from my roles.

At first, I stayed up all night and slept most of the day. I thought a lot, took long walks on the beach. That was when I sat with the seagull. I thanked God for each day, meditated and read.

I was not afraid of taking large blocks of time for myself. But I was afraid that by not working, by dropping out of the world, I was admitting I was dying. I felt that teaching was keeping me alive.

The semester away from school started off like a race to get to the fundamental core—who I am and where my life force comes from—so I could use it creatively. I put myself on the line again by staying by myself. I knew that if I had just a few months to live, I didn't want to spend them teaching piano.

I wanted to spend them doing these interior things. At last, I had to answer that question: What would fill your whole day with joy?

During that period, I learned more about love. Learning to love, even to say the word, is a difficult thing. My mother was angry with me over an incident and I was very hurt. How can she be so angry, I wondered, when she doesn't know how long I'll be here? The next morning I dialed my parents' phone.

"I love you," I said as soon as my mother answered. "And I want to stay in communication with you."

There was a stunned silence. I hadn't said such a thing since I was a very young child. She began to cry.

In November, Tyler was laid off his job because of company financial troubles. We didn't worry about it much. Money just isn't that important anymore.

On December 7, 1987, I celebrated my 31st birthday. The doctors had predicted I wouldn't see 30. Three days later I went to see my oncologist. I often wake up on those mornings depressed and discouraged. Going to see the doctor is always a setup for maybe feeling worse. I've learned to put on extra emotional padding on those days, and not to take in a suggestion from an authority figure if I don't agree with it.

The oncologist said I looked better, that I'd put on weight and looked more energetic than ever.

"I'm not sure there's much for me to do," he said shrugging his shoulders. "I never know if you'll do what I tell you to, anyway."

He took a few tests and I walked toward the door.

"You'll really have to tell me what you're doing," he said. "Someday, when we have the time ..."

I think frequently about those lists that I made during the summer of 1986. The "live" list filled a page and a half. The "die" list filled a page. If I had made those lists before my illness, the "die" list would have been the longer.

After this fall, after my time alone and my time with the seagull, I would never consider making such a list. There is no reason to die. And there is only one reason to live: to love.

EPILOGUE

Julie died in July 1988, almost three years after refusing to have a bone marrow transplant, and two years after the medical crisis that caused doctors to predict "two weeks to live."

Before her death, Julie asked her oncologist to discuss her case for this book. He refused.

Julie's homeopathic doctor, Dr. Ahmed N. Currim of Norwalk, Connecticut, said Julie had several crises during her illness.

"Her recovery from these crises was completely unexpected from a medical point of view," Currim said. "All her doctors believe she lived several years longer than expected."

Many people in the traditional medical community never accepted Julie's decision not to have the bone marrow transplant, believing she should cling to life no matter what the cost. But Tyler said Julie never regretted her decision, even on the day of her death.

"To exercise those medical options would have been one way of choosing," Tyler said three months after Julie's death. "But Julie wished not to make her choices based on fear. In her own heart, she could not see the bone marrow transplant as other than a resort based on fear, fear of

death. Julie wanted to face her fears, follow a course of self-love and make her choices based on that love.

"The point of taking responsibility for yourself—and accepting all the possibilities that come from that—is how she made the decision not to have the transplant. She made the decision to live as fully as possible while she was alive, without dramatic medical intervention, so that she would always be the one directing her life, despite the illness. If that meant dying, that was acceptable to her.

"Like the bird she watched, Julie made a powerful statement, surrendering to death as a natural culmination of life. Julie's display of faith was the most peaceful thing I have ever witnessed. Her death was horrible, but it was perfect.

"All summer long, I know now, she was preparing to die. But she protected me from that knowledge until the last few days. She asked to be taken to the hospital, the first time she had been in a hospital since her diagnosis, I think in order to make things easier for the rest of us.

"She died three days later with very little struggle. In our fear, we believe death is a loss, a giving in. From Julie's three-year search, she learned how to join life and death into a unity, and achieved a special healing of the spirit in the process.

"So her death in the hospital was a smooth progression, gentle and loving, exactly the way she would do something, a perfect expression of herself. To watch her those last few days was to witness someone totally at peace, totally without fear. Her faith was complete.

"This was the miracle."

Joe Ayoob

INTRODUCTION

In June 1975, Joe Ayoob settled into an all-night poker game on the Amtrak special out of Boston headed for Texas. He was playing for keeps, gambling for his life.

Behind Joe, back in Boston, was a doctor who had given up treating a brain tumor metastasized from lung cancer. Calling the cancer incurable, the doctor predicted Joe's death within six months.

But waiting for Joe down in Texas was an off-beat oncologist who believed Joe could "imagine" his cancer out of existence. He called his technique "visualization."

With no conventional medical alternatives left to try, Joe boarded the Amtrak special and played poker on the ride south, wondering what hand fate would deal him down in Texas.

Joe's Story

Three years earlier, when the cancer first appeared, I was selling encyclopedias out in California, smoking lots of marijuana, and living pretty high and fast.

It sounds funny: selling encyclopedias. But I liked it. I liked it at first, anyway. I was so shy and so lonely, and knocking on doors to talk about books was a good way to get some company. I loved walking into people's homes like that, sitting down over coffee in a living room with someone and having them listen when I told about the encyclopedia.

Maybe that was the first time in my life anybody wanted to hear what I had to say. I was so good at the door-to-door stuff that the encyclopedia company gave me a trip to Curaçao and made me team manager.

But by 1972, the year the cancer came, I didn't like the work anymore. I got tired of talking to strangers I would never see again, and I started to feel like I just couldn't knock on one more door. As my attitude got worse, more and more people started slamming doors in my face. I was hardly selling anything. I wasn't making any money. But I sure was doing a lot of drugs.

The idea of suicide started out almost like a game. What if suicide were the only way out? Would I have the courage to do it? How would I do it? What would it feel like? The game became a mental obsession. I turned over the possibilities, the methods, and the results in my mind, hour after hour. Maybe suicide was the only option left in a pointless world.

Back in Boston, dragging more than ever, I had a checkup at the Veterans Administration Hospital. Lung cancer, the doctor announced. Five more years to live. That's what he told me, anyway. To my mother, he said: six months at the most. After exploratory surgery, the surgeons cut out one-fourth of the left lung. I took only one treatment from an experimental chemotherapy protocol and refused the rest. I did have radiation. Lots of radiation.

Living in California, I had been thinking about death all the time, imagining the feeling, but when that doctor said I had only a few years left, I cried. I cried a lot. I didn't want my chance at living taken away. It's different when it's not your decision anymore. I didn't even know the doctor told my mother I had only six months.

Then, a few days later, I started feeling the incredibility of the thing. It just didn't make any sense to get to 33—and then die. It just didn't make any sense. I hadn't gotten started yet. I was just getting over the obstacle of being young. I wanted to scream to heaven.

After the surgery I started writing, doing some philosophical trips. I know it sounds strange, but it was a nice summer because I started to get a handle on what was going on, on where things were leading. I started feeling more positive about myself.

I don't know how, exactly, that happened. I know I created good feelings in order to keep the bad feelings aside. And that helped. I also started reading books that told about the power a person has, that everything is possible and that everything you can imagine can be achieved.

I came to a decision about death: It scared the shit out of me. I didn't want any part of it. Before, in California, I had only been playing with the idea. That summer, I said to myself: "I'm too young to die. I'm not going to die, so I may as well get started living."

See, I hadn't really accomplished anything. I was terrified of death, and I felt there would be less fear of dying if I had accomplished something. I wasn't sure exactly what that meant. It took me several years to get a handle on what I wanted to accomplish and how to go about it.

I don't want you to think this is easy, that you wake up and say, "I don't want cancer," and it's gone. Even today, I'm not willing to say how much of my healing came from me and how much came from the doctors.

My own change took years. There were lots of physical setbacks, lots and lots of despairing days and weeks and months. At first, I just sat back and expected the doctors to do everything. I was the cancer "victim" and their job was to do something about it.

I was so into that role of patient—I know you won't believe this—that I kept chain smoking. The whole time I was in and out of the hospital for the radiation, while the cancer kept growing and metastasizing, I kept smoking cigarettes. And I never did any of the other things some people do, like eating macrobiotic food or special vegetarian food, meditation and doing exercises like tai chi. I didn't do a lot of intensive introspection.

After the lung surgery, the cancer metastasized to my brain. It's a common route, from the lung to the brain. It could have gone there, or it could have gone to the liver. Once again, I had a lot of radiation. No chemotherapy, just radiation. The chemotherapy was experimental, and they kept telling me that it killed the good cells along with the bad cells. I just didn't want it.

Then, after all that, suddenly my eye went. The muscle was gone. I couldn't control it anymore, and I couldn't see anything. At that point I was pretty tired. The doctors had done everything they could. They just didn't have anything more left. After the third radiation treatment, the one for the eye, I got discouraged with so much radiation. It left so much scar tissue.

I decided the rest was up to me. I had to start making the decisions myself. I'd been reading books about the power of the human mind and I decided to visualize myself well. I did something I'd never done before. I wrote a letter to all my friends and asked them to visualize along with me, every day from 12 noon until five minutes after. It wasn't much of an effort. I only wrote eight letters; I didn't have that many friends. I don't even know if they did it, but it was important to me. I imagined all my friends imagining me well.

I did other stuff, too. I tried going to a faith healer. I stood in line in front of a Philadelphia church for hours, just waiting to get in. But she turned out to be a fake.

When my eye went, that's when I decided to head out to Texas to the Simonton Clinic. I didn't have any money to pay for it, but they said to come out. I don't even know how I got the money for the train ride. I guess I borrowed it or something. I was living on a VA disability pension and was real poor.

So I took the Amtrak. On the way down, I hooked up with a couple of guys going down to Vegas. The three of us had a ball. They never knew I had cancer or why I was going to Texas. We just played cards all night long. I don't normally do stuff like that, but I figured I may as well get into the game of chance for all I was worth. I didn't lose any money, but I didn't win any, either.

Then, when I got to Texas, I just broke down. I cried and cried, but I was determined to get everything I could out of that time. Seeing other people sick like me helped, that and doing a lot of group therapy.

The two weeks at the clinic were the high point of my life. Still are. It wasn't just the group therapy, although that was important. It was the camaraderie. People were caring and supportive; everyone was so close in such a short time. We lived at a hotel close to the clinic and got together to cook at night. It was a community thing, a group effort, a sharing.

That was different for me. We were all together for the same reasons. I'd never done that before, shared with others like that and enjoyed being with them. We had something very important in common.

The day I got to the clinic, we had a personality test. The test was supposed to be about self-image. I did poorly, very poorly. The test measures self-worth and acceptance, and I'll tell you, over the past decade since I left the Simontons', I've taken several more. My scores keep getting better and better.

Actually doing the visualization was difficult for me.

Somehow, I think the acceptance I felt from other people at the clinic was more important than the visualizing.

In California, visiting my sister for a few weeks, I decided to take the eye patch off. I didn't really do it as a test or anything. I wanted to drive her car. When I took the patch off, I could see perfectly. I was feeling pretty good, coming in from Texas, so I wasn't surprised.

I haven't had any problems with the cancer since then. It just never came back. But I did have to go into the hospital a few years ago because of a stroke. The radiation for the brain tumor caused massive scar tissue, which in turn caused a stroke. While I was in the hospital this time, I wasn't worried. I knew by then that I wasn't going to die in any hospital, that I would recover from whatever happened.

One doctor, a radiation doctor, used to say to me, "Such a miracle." He couldn't believe I was still alive. Part of it is just being stubborn: You're not going to take what's dished out. I just wouldn't see the truth that others saw: my death.

Now the doctors say it must have been the radiation. I don't think it was one or the other; I think the credit has to be shared. I would never say my part was 100 percent. But I did something. I discovered who I was. I discovered I wanted to play the piano, be a jazz musician. And that's what I did.

I've discovered a side of me that's very disciplined and controlled. Every day for the past seven years, I've practiced four or five hours a day. At first, learning was hard. But I stayed with it, kept playing, because I knew that was what I had to do.

Music is a religious experience for me. If anything is spiritual, music is. Music is a deep part of my nature. Life without it would be senseless. I gave myself a sense of purpose and meaning, but I didn't start playing for that reason.

I really had no choice: The music owns me, I don't own it. I was refusing it, and there's a certain price to be paid for refusing part of yourself. I guess that sounds romantic, but as the years go by I understand that more and more clearly.

A lot of people who are ill ask me for suggestions about what they should do. I can't tell you specific stuff, or doctors you should go to, or what kind of food you should eat.

But I can tell you one very important thing that you should know about me: I overcame it. It can be done. There's nothing special about me. "Hope" is just a human quality that we all share. Maybe it was the luck of the draw. Maybe I just got sick, and then I just got better. That's what some people say, especially the doctors.

But I don't believe that. I know why I got cancer when I was 33, and I know why I'm better now. I had a miserable childhood. I never grew up with anybody around me and I went to boarding school when I was three years old. I went to a Catholic boarding school with a very big nun. The more she hit me, the more I rebelled. I never learned social skills, and to minimize that, I spent time by myself. I stayed alone most of the time. My mother remarried when I was nine, and I didn't get along with her new husband very well. It wasn't his fault, he just didn't know what to do with a kid like me. I quit school in the tenth grade and started working. I joined the army, and after the army I started working at a bank, opening letters.

This is the kind of person who gets cancer, who can't express himself, who gets beaten down. I never really liked myself, and I never really helped myself until I got sick.

Then I found out that I wanted to be alive. I didn't want to kick off, like I thought I did. I realized I had never given myself a chance. Until I began playing music seriously, I never had anything to live for, anything outside of myself to keep me motivated and interested in life.

This is important: It's not the decisions that you make about how to get better. It's what's behind those decisions that's important. The outcome always depends on how you feel about yourself. For the most part, I made bad decisions about living my life. I didn't do many of the things for myself that I should have done. I wasn't living my life the way I really wanted to.

The illness changed the way I felt about myself. I started making different decisions. I didn't turn the corner right away, it wasn't a sharp right turn. But I did do it.

Now I love to play the piano. I just can't believe what kind of beauty there is in the world. I always played the piano, but it was haphazard before. I never had the discipline to work. I don't have any money; I'm still poor, living on my disability pension. But I'm doing the thing that is important to me.

This next thing is, I have to start playing for other people. You can guess, by now, how hard that will be for me. But that's part of the decision I made about my life when I was still sick, that I would learn music and give it to others. I played for a group of people at my teacher's house a few weeks ago. That was the first time. It was successful in that I played my best. I put myself out there and didn't hang back. I opened myself up, and had fun doing it.

EPILOGUE

Because Joe was treated by a succession of Veterans Administration doctors, none of whom remains on the staff at Boston's VA Hospital, interviewing doctors about Joe's case was not possible.

But Joe was able to present his complete medical records, which remain on file at the hospital. The records are massively thick, with paper filed mostly between September 1973, the time of the initial diagnosis, and November 1978, the final period of hospitalization for treatment of his stroke.

Records indicate that in September 1973, Joe underwent a "left upper lobectomy" due to a "poorly differentiated carcinoma of the lung."

In June 1974, the records say, a "brain scan was pos-

itive in the left parietal region," and radiation was prescribed.

A year later came a third incident, "right orbital metastasis" in the brain. On September 11, 1975, the patient was given "palliative radiotherapy to his right retro-orbital region. The recent CT scans reveal evidence of a space occupying lesion which resulted in proptosis of the right eyeball."

Subsequently, following Joe's visit to Texas and California, the records indicate a substantial change.

The next tests reveal "clinical and angiographic resolution of the orbital mass." After that, except for the period during the stroke, the records are consistent: "Currently doing well with stable weight." "No evidence of acute disease." "No evidence of metastasis."

Charles Yellowley

INTRODUCTION

In the windowless, disorienting environment of a Toronto intensive care ward, Charles Yellowley faced an agonizing crossroad. Doctors had just removed one tumor from the back of his skull but hadn't found the source of the illness that still threatened his life. From either side of his bed came the sounds of dying patients and grieving families, accentuating the bleakness of his own situation.

A lifetime spent seeking and achieving career and financial success hadn't prepared him to deal with this desolation. He had invested his intellect, passion, and family feeling in the high-pressured world of television news, and now that world seemed closed to him. He had no idea what the future could offer him, or whether he had a future to consider.

Slowly, tentatively, for the first time as an adult, Charles reached out for human help, and found it. Medical treatment coordinated by a sympathetic oncologist kept the illness at bay. An experimental cancer-support group helped him achieve a sense of possibility. And, at a critical moment, Charles found a way back to the religious tradition he had feared was lost to him forever.

Charles' Story

I live in a condominium, high above Lake Ontario. Every once in a while, an errant seagull flies into one of my picture windows, smashes into the glass with a loud crash, and falls 15 floors to the ground below.

When cancer happened to me, that's how I felt. I had always been a winner, flying higher and harder and faster than anyone else. Then one day I hit something that I couldn't beat. The fall was a hard one.

At 47, I had worked my way to the top in a ruthless world—television news broadcasting. And I did it by myself, too. I wasn't one of those young kids who gets handed stuff by a rich uncle. I started at the bottom and worked hard.

I grew up in a very conservative small town in Ontario. My father died just before I was born, and my mother never remarried and never talked about him. My father was a great mystery figure, and I grew up a lonely boy raised by a very religious Irish Catholic widow. For as far back as I can remember, music and community life were a part of me. I sang in the church choir as a boy, went to a Jesuit school, and as soon as I finished school started working as a disc jockey on the local radio station.

Doing country-and-western shows, saying the same things over and over again on the radio, became very boring very quickly. When a job covering the local news opened up, I grabbed it—chasing fire engines in a radio station van. I married and took a radio job in Montreal, where I covered the separatist bombings during the 1960s. When my company launched a local television station, I moved into television news, working at first in black-and-white.

It was a sensational way of life at first, covering Montreal's Expo '67 World's Fair and visits by the Shah of Iran, Charles de Gaulle, Lyndon Johnson. I got to meet prime ministers and kings. But eventually even this became boring. As a reporter, you're not making the command decisions. Someone else decides whether and when and how your story runs.

Someone else decides the content and the length. Someone else decides the importance of your work in the scheme of the nightly news broadcast.

So I became a producer of the news and ultimately became the executive producer of daily news for the CTV Television Network Ltd., Canada's privately owned national network. The pressure of that position, coveted and prestigious as it is, is tremendous. We compete nightly with the Canadian Broadcasting Company, the publicly owned network. At CTV, we started out with a much smaller staff and had to work much harder with much less money to produce a competitive nightly news program.

As the producer of the national news, I was making up a broadcast "front page" every day, coordinating our reporters around the world and our bureaus across Canada, getting a package of goodies ready for "11 o'clock straight up" every night. It was a constant wrangle. You fear making mistakes that will be seen immediately by 2 million people. You fear making mistakes that will cause lawsuits and cost the network big bucks. You fear making even minor timing mistakes that will irritate advertisers and lose the network advertising income.

The deadlines come at you without a letup from early in the morning, when you start deciding on stories for that night's broadcast, until the broadcast is over. Then you come in the next morning, and it starts all over again. You're working five, six, seven days a week, coming home late, never having time for any kind of life outside the network.

Inside I was filled with despair. Here I was succeeding beyond the wildest dreams of my youth, and I was miserable. I had this perfectionist personality: No matter how hard I worked, I was never good enough. Good enough to please myself, that is. I always saw more mistakes, more imperfections, more room for improvement in each broadcast than anyone else. After a difficult production, I would try to reward myself by buying a new suit, a new car, something nice. But it never worked. I was looking for a reward I would never get, trying to buy something that had to come from inside.

And if you come home to a marriage that isn't working— and mine wasn't—everything in your life is stress. After a number of years I began to realize that I couldn't keep this up forever. But I didn't know what to do. The company had become the only family I really had. I devoted my whole life to this high-stress business and had no friends outside of the world of television and news broadcasting. I was an emotional cripple.

I knew the nerve-wracking stress could kill me—I had watched several colleagues die from heart disease and cancer by this time—but I wasn't doing anything about it. Sitting quietly and contemplating life was just not a value much emphasized in my world. I was stressed out by my job, unhappy in my marriage, and obviously ignoring inner needs. But in the action-oriented world of television news, you just don't ask for time off to contemplate existence. In fact I was such a private person that most of my friends at work didn't know for many years that my wife had left me. I knew about their personal lives, but they never knew the most basic details of mine.

I wouldn't stop my world and take time off, and finally my body did it for me. In 1984, while I was coordinating coverage of a national election, I started having terrible headaches. I frequently flew into temper tantrums, yelling at waiters and service-station attendants. I began to have trouble walking properly and enunciating clearly. While friends would drink doubles at lunch, I would order Perrier, fearful that otherwise my slurred speech would make people think I was drunk.

I could still conduct staff meetings and engineer news coverage. But when the meetings were over I was careful to let others leave first, rather than stumble or lurch out of the room ahead of them.

Finally, my doctor ordered a CT scan. I went to the hospital for the scan and then went off directly to a meeting of communications staff to discuss election coverage details. Around 5 p.m., the neurologist called the network.

"Could you come and see me on your way to work tomorrow morning?" he asked.

I knew something was up, or he wouldn't have asked for a first-thing-in-the-morning meeting.

"There's a large mass in the brain," he said the next morning. "The neurosurgeon is waiting to talk to you in town right now. Go and see him immediately. But don't drive. Take a taxi."

After a brief taxi ride, I found the neurosurgeon was, indeed, waiting for me.

"There's a tumor there," he said, "growing larger every day. That's what's causing the pain. I can operate and remove it."

"Well," I answered, "when do you want to do this?"

"How's tomorrow morning," he said, not making it a question. "You can just stay here now and get checked in immediately. My nurse will help you."

I told him I was in the middle of coordinating TV news coverage of a national election.

"This tumor has to come out or you'll be dead in six weeks," he said. "I want you admitted now. The surgery has to be tomorrow morning."

The hospital room wasn't quite ready, an orderly told me. So I left for a few hours to take care of a few details and to go home to pack a suitcase. While I was gone, the hospital staff had hit the panic button and begun searching frantically for me all over the city.

"We've just given this guy some bad news," they told my boss, the network vice-president. "And now he's disappeared."

They put me on the ninth floor, the neurosurgery floor, and my sister came to spend the night with me. We spent most of those hours before the surgery talking, mostly about the loose ends of my life. What a hell of a mess: A frenetic life-style, a broken marriage, and now a brain tumor. We talked about my future, assuming I had one.

The next morning they dug a three-centimeter-by-five-centimeter tumor out of my head. It was lodged between the skull and the back of the brain, and pressure from it was affecting motor coordination and speech.

That was June 8, 1984. When I woke up, I was in the hospital's Fellini Room. That's what I called it. They called it the intensive care ward for neurological patients. I think it was designed by studying the latest techniques for brainwashing and mental torture. No windows. No phones. No newspapers. No clocks or televisions or information sources of any kind.

That's just how they wanted it, like a science fiction spaceship. Nurses sit at the foot of your bed and take notes constantly. Behind you are masses and masses of life-support systems. Hourly, someone wakes you to see if your brain is still working.

"What's your name?" the nurse asks, tapping your toes with a pencil, or "What day is it?"

Mind-bending is the only way to describe it. I developed systems to tell what time of day it was. If the nurses were talking about an evening with their boyfriends, I decided it must be morning. If I was offered tea to drink, I decided it must be afternoon. Having developed this system, I once had a terrible temper tantrum when they offered me tea but brought me coffee. Was I crazy? Or were they trying to confuse me?

There was no privacy. The nurses had to be able to see us

constantly, to monitor our machines. Nothing separated one patient from another except a curtain that could be pulled shut if a patient was having difficulty—or was dying. I listened first to the patient on one side of me die. Then, to the crying of a young wife on the other side as her husband died.

I listened to a doctor convince a husband to pull the plug on his wife, who was brain dead. I listened to the husband agonize over the decision, sure he was murdering his wife. Death became real, not something to be reported. I watched it happen around me over and over again. Then I heard the surgeon tell me my turn could be just around the corner.

I wasn't even sure I was alive. Once I got up and walked around and spotted a newspaper. No one was on guard at the nurses' desk. I grabbed the paper, went back to my bed, and pulled the curtains around me so no one could see what I was doing.

Then I turned to the obituaries. I looked up my name, to see if I had died the night before.

I remember opening my eyes and seeing my sister.

"Thank God," I thought. "There's my sister. I must be alive." But I touched her, just to make sure.

After a few days, the neurosurgeon came for a short visit, accompanied by his minions.

"You're doing very well," he said to me. "The operation was a success. The only problem was, the tumor was malignant. And it was a secondary tumor," meaning—I found out later—that the doctors hadn't touched the source of the illness.

For the first time in my life, the high flier was knocked low. Not just low, but knocked totally out of the running. In 48 hours, I had gone from running a national news network to being asked if I could spell my own name. Words were my profession, yet I didn't understand the language spoken in that room. What's a metastasis? In a room full of constant crisis, no one had time to stop and explain things to me.

The Fellini Room was an end, and it was a beginning. I

started to change. I started to understand that I needed help. I started to ask for help.

"I can't do this by myself," I said to one person. "I need someone to help me get through this."

Never, never before in my life had I asked for such a thing. Never, never had I said I couldn't do something on my own. Surrounded by death in the Fellini Room, recognizing the possibility—even likelihood—of my own death, I knew I needed to develop some deeper level of understanding.

During those eight days in intensive care, a priest stopped to talk.

"I don't think I'm worth your trouble," I told him. "I think I'm probably ineligible."

So we talked about hockey. There were, by that time, so many bricks in the wall between myself and the church. I hadn't attended mass or confession for so long. I didn't like a lot of the priests I had met since childhood, the kind who drank too much wine or kept girlfriends. And the church had changed so much, allowing meat on Fridays, saying the mass in English. And the church had annulled my marriage without consulting me. My wife, my ex-wife, informed me after the fact.

I was raised in the old regime, where sin is serious business. I figured I was just unworthy by now, so the priest and I didn't talk about religion and he didn't try to bless me.

From the Fellini Room, I went to a private hospital room. In many ways this was worse. I could see the real world from my window, and people sent cards and flowers from the out-side. But I was separated forever from that world now, by a barrier that could never be recrossed. The world I could see from the window wasn't for me. I was stuck in this room with a problem: I had this fatal illness.

The neurosurgeon handed me over to an oncologist, who would oversee future radiation and chemotherapy treatments. The first time I met him, he sat down in a chair and looked up at me in the hospital bed. I knew I would get along with him.

But I kept having this feeling at first that he was testing me, seeing if I was worth the trouble, seeing if I would survive. He explained the illness and treatments.

"We're not going to cure you," he said, "but we're going to improve the quality of your life."

At some point, we had a further conversation, in which I pushed him to discuss longevity.

"Will I still be talking to you in a year?" I asked him.

"Yes."

"In two years?"

"Probably."

"In three years?"

He hesitated.

"Well, if we're still friends."

Later we had another conversation.

"Ninety percent of people with small-cell carcinoma don't survive," I said.

"Ten percent do," he replied. "Why not be part of that group?"

Doctors initially diagnosed my cancer as a small-cell or "oat-cell" carcinoma and believed the brain tumor was a secondary tumor. Eventually I learned that small-cell carcinoma is a cancer usually starting in the lungs. Once metastasized to the brain, this cancer carries very, very low survival rates. I learned that a secondary tumor means the original tumor started elsewhere, and that metastasis means that the cancerous cells have traveled through the body.

The strange thing about this cancer was that I had given up smoking many years earlier and no trace of cancer was ever found in my lungs. The doctors were mystified.

Coming out of the Fellini Room was a little like being reborn, like leaving the womb. Again I began asking for help. Suddenly, everything familiar was destroyed. How do you pick up the pieces? What do you do next? Why didn't I die?

"I really need some answers," I told a social worker—a

warm and comforting woman who became a special ally during this period. "I haven't got a handle on any of this. I'm not in control for the first time in my life. I need someone to come and tell me why I was chosen as a cancer patient."

She arranged for several sessions with a hospital psychiatrist. But that went nowhere. He was young and had little familiarity himself with death. He asked a lot of questions and got a lot of answers from me, but I was still left with just questions.

Then the social worker mentioned that an experimental group had started at the Ontario Cancer Institute, a group of cancer patients led by Alastair Cunningham, a psychologist and immunologist at the institute. At that time, only 20 patients could participate, and you had to have a personal interview with Alastair to qualify.

When I went there to talk, Alastair really reached out, listening carefully and offering real responses and even a few answers.

"What do you want from the group?" he asked.

"I want something like Alcoholics Anonymous," I answered, "where I can sit around with other cancer patients under your direction and learn how to get a handle on this. I really want to meet some other guys who, like me, were just shot down in midair for no apparent reason."

We talked for a long time, and finally he accepted me. I had returned to my apartment to live, but a bad reaction to chemotherapy put me back in the hospital. The night of the first meeting, I told the ward nurses I had to leave for a few hours, but they refused to let me out.

"I must go," I said. "It's vitally important that I go to this meeting. I just can't miss it."

Finally, the nurses called my oncologist, who agreed that I should go.

I loved the first meeting. To talk to other patients, to sit quietly in a group like that and not feel like a freak, or that everyone was feeling sorry for me, was so important.

Alastair told us to close our eyes, and he talked about what we would do in the group. He explained relaxation exercises and told us we would be doing mental imagery, visualization, and mantras. We all sat and chanted "ooommmmm" together.

Truthfully, I thought the mantras were silly as hell. And I thought a lot of this other stuff was mumbo jumbo. I wasn't used to trying to relax and thought visualizing a white light was a waste of time.

I kept coming back to the meetings, though, because I valued the friendships forming in the group. Sharing the link of cancer with these other men and women kept me going during a period when I wasn't sure I wanted to keep going.

The folks at the hospital saved my life physically, but all the way along I was an emotional basket case. Alastair and the group saved my life mentally, by helping me understand and open myself up. I think you really can wish yourself dead, and that's what I was doing before I started that group.

And I learned, despite my original attitude, that the tools taught by Alastair really could help me cope. I gained a spiritual sort of energy by meditation. And I did learn to visualize a white light entering and flooding my body. That light can overcome the despair and utter hopelessness I still feel from time to time.

But I couldn't get into a lot of the John Lennon–type stuff. One night I was sitting in the back of the group when these people in orange robes came dancing in. I was pretty embarrassed. And I was pretty confused.

"How firm is this guy?" I wondered to myself about Alastair. "Will it work if I only accept part of this stuff, or do you have to go for the whole bit, like the Jesuits wanted?"

One night we were sitting there all chanting "ooommmm" and I decided to open up.

"You're shoveling up all this stuff from Katmandu," I said. "But I think I'm a little too old for this now. I'm an Irish Catholic."

I'd reached the stage where my own religion was creeping back, and I didn't need the swamis and the gurus. Religion reentered my life through a back door held open by Alastair Cunningham, swami and group leader extraordinaire.

I still had very uncomfortable feelings about the Catholic church. There was the terrible fear about being unacceptable to my maker. I was obviously unacceptable to my grandparents and parents, because they all died and left me. I was unacceptable to my wife, because she walked out.

So I was worried about being unacceptable to God. You build up all these bricks in the wall, and I despaired of ever breaking through. I hadn't been to church for many years, and in the midst of a high-pressured career it had become acceptable not to bother. Then lightning strikes in your brain.

"Oh, I'm sorry, God," you say. "Now I need your help."

I didn't feel right about that. And I also knew it wouldn't work. As a boy in Kingston, I learned from the ultraconservative Catholic church that God is not very kind, but he might listen to you if you play the game his way. I hadn't been playing by the rules.

"The devil walks the streets of this parish," Father O'Neil had warned. "And if he gets you and you're not in a state of grace, you'll burn in the fires of hell."

Well, the devil had certainly got me at last, with a giant zap to the brain. And I was certainly not in a state of grace.

I was also, truth to tell, angry at the church. The marriage annulment wasn't the only thing. In the church, in my own cathedral in Kingston, they tore down the beautiful majestic marble altars because, under Vatican II changes, the priests celebrating the mass prepare the host while facing the congregation. I was afraid to go to church because all the prayers I had learned in Latin as a boy were now in English, and I might not be able to speak them correctly.

All that winter, 1984–1985, I sat brooding in my apartment. There were endless gray days with the snow falling. It got to the point where I talked to the plants and the furniture. One day I had a big fight with the vacuum cleaner.

On one of those days, a friend called to say his parish priest would be making visits near my apartment.

"Would you like this guy to come see you?" my friend asked.

I was so lonely, I figured I may as well just have it out with the guy. I figured he'd probably tell me I was worthless, or that I had to spend three years in sackcloth and ashes before being allowed back in the church.

"You've been brought up in the old way," the priest said, after I told him my fears. "There's no reason for you to carry this around. Look, it's different now. The rules, the Jesuitical discipline, that's for training kids. Look again at your religion and you'll find something different as an adult.

"You walk into a garden and pick the flowers that you want," he told me. "That's what your religion is, a garden where you sit when you want to, or when you need to."

He brought me around to believing that I could reestablish some connection with the church. Before, I had assumed I was having a satellite transmission problem, that I had been beaming up messages that weren't being accepted.

The priest recited the prayers set aside for the extremely ill. He anointed me with holy oil, on my forehead, on my lips, on both hands.

"For all the thoughts, words, and deeds: All is now forgiven," he said. Then he left.

I was jolted by this. Call it symbolic. Call it real. Whatever. I became again a member in good standing. I cried and cried. I sobbed and slept. It was dark when I woke up, and my mind felt happy.

Since that day, I have had a more peaceful kind of courage, a courage backed up by a sense of something greater than me. I've had several recurrences of secondary tumors. My renewed faith doesn't lessen the burden of those tumors, but it does bring me greater calm and less loneliness. And I believe those changes have helped me fight the cancer successfully.

EPILOGUE

Over the past four years, Charles has had five recurrences of his illness. Most have been in his spine, none have been in the brain, and none have been as severe as the initial tumor.

He has kept up his relationship with the cancer support group, and has continued to use the tools learned in the group to help calm his fears and control his depression.

He has continued his road back to the Catholic church, attends services regularly, and has received several more sacraments, which hold deepening significance for him. ,

His sixth recurrence, in the fall of 1988, caused a partial but very frightening paralysis, including an inability to walk unassisted. But by December, after radiation eradicated the tumor, Charles was again vigorously striding the walking trails along the bluffs overlooking Lake Ontario.

None of this, he insists, would have been possible were it not for his medical team, the cancer support group, and the priest who visited his apartment that gray winter day.

The course of Charles' disease is extremely unusual, as he has successfully endured so many recurrences, said oncologist Robert Myers of Toronto's St. Michael's Hospital.

"Despite these well-documented episodes of spinal cord lesions, he's still very fit. His continued responses and mobility have been a bit surprising but very gratifying," Myers said.

After removal of the brain tumor, he said, pathologists diagnosed Charles as having small-cell carcinoma, also called "oat cell," metastasized to the brain. This extremely aggressive cancer most frequently begins in the lungs.

However, since no lung lesion was ever located and since the course of the disease has not followed a typical "oat-cell" pattern, Myers said, the cancer may be a medulloblastoma, a somewhat less aggressive disease, much more common in children than in adults.

"Mr. Yellowley has responded quite predictably to our radiation treatments," Myers said. "What's unusual is to be fit after so many recurrences. While I do not think the support group has had any effect on his health, I do believe the group has helped him deal with his anger at his illness, at having to give up his work. He is much calmer and more relaxed, much more accepting of what's happened."

Smadar Levin

INTRODUCTION

In 1987, at Christmastime, Smadar Levin flew from Boston to Brazil, where she spent more than a month living and praying in a mountain spiritual community. Despite her very advanced cancer, Smadar celebrated several religious festivals with the community, dancing through the night. During those rituals, Smadar says, she experienced her own death and the presence of God.

Smadar's Story

I refuse to become a cancer patient. I am a human being—who also has cancer. This often makes treating me difficult for my doctors and sometimes makes loving me painful for friends and family, who want to protect me.

But I believe this attitude—this search for God and spirit, and this insistence on living in the world given us—has kept me alive. Statistics, if you're interested in that kind of thing, say I should have died a decade ago. But new events in life keep renewing my commitment, revealing new pathways in my search for understanding. I believe my personal and spiritual work have both minimized the effects of the illness and enhanced my medical treatments.

People get cancer for different reasons, and we can't always know what those reasons are. At some point I started to believe that perhaps my soul chose this to learn some important lessons. I must add, though, that I certainly don't think this is true for everybody.

For me, cancer has resulted in a major shift in my perception of the world. I began my cancer experience as a primarily left-brained person: rational, separatist, self-sufficient. Born in Israel, I was raised in the Jewish culture, but without a strong emphasis on God and spirit. I was an atheist and thought God was just a culturally convenient belief system, created to make people feel good.

"It might help you to believe in God," my husband, Mike, said to me when I first became ill.

"I don't need a crutch," I answered. Silly me.

I have spent my life looking for answers, looking for the truth. At first, I believed the truth lay in science. Cancer has taught me that science is one of many truths, one of many levels of reality, which finally integrate to form the ultimate reality, blending the scientific into the spiritual. Science is a way of thinking about our three-dimensional world. Spirit is a way of understanding dimensions that science cannot penetrate.

In 1973, when I was 27, my Israeli husband and I came to America, hoping to earn our doctorates. I was invited to enter Harvard's department of psychology, but my husband was not invited to join the program of his choice. While I loved the New England climate, the new culture and new language, and the intellectual vitality of Harvard, my husband's experience was different. Without the hoped-for doctoral program, he felt adrift in the new culture, and spent his days in our North Cambridge apartment watching television. We were living on two completely different wavelengths. One day I came home to find him packing to return to Israel.

My husband's departure was saddening, but not devastating, as we hadn't been getting along well. But it added another degree of stress to an already stressful year. Despite my exhilaration, working hard in a demanding program and living in a new culture were difficult. I'm a somatizer: I work my emotions out in my body. Piling the stress of that first year on top of a lifelong depression and lack of self-esteem, perhaps it's not surprising that I developed breast cancer.

Just about a year after my arrival in the United States, I felt an olive-sized lump in my left breast. My second husband-to-be, Mike, and I had spent a fall foliage weekend in New Hampshire with friends. I had been very depressed all fall; that weekend was particularly difficult for me. When we got back home, I just put my hand on my left breast and felt the lump. I was 28, never practiced breast self-examination, and never thought about cancer. But semiconsciously, I knew what it was.

A doctor at the university's health service, a woman who was a friend of mine, examined me. Both of us were heavily invested emotionally in the lump being benign, and it did have all the characteristics of nonmalignancy: It was soft, movable, and painful. I had no family history of cancer. A negative mammogram confirmed what we wanted to hear.

As my friend, the doctor didn't really want to diagnose the lump. We decided to wait and watch. She denied and I denied, and we just kind of sat on it until my family said something. My mother, especially, was insistent when I visited her, asking me at least to have a family friend, a surgeon, look at it.

"It looks benign," he agreed after the examination, "but why take any chances? Why not just have it out?"

The cautious approach made sense, so I arranged to have the lump removed on an outpatient basis, still feeling confident that nothing was wrong. So I was quite unprepared for a phone call from the operating doctor's nurse.

"The doctor wants to see you because the cells are malignant," she said.

She told me just like that, over the phone with no preparation. After a few moments of shock, I ran out of the computer room, where I was working, down the hall to the office of a friend, barely able to talk. My friend called Mike to come and get me.

"Cancer," I thought. "This is it. I have cancer."

Hearing the word spoken, speaking it yourself, is like crossing a magical line from one life into another. I'd had the lump for seven months and had known the possibilities for those same seven months. But a possibility is so different from a reality.

I denied the diagnosis. I started thinking there was a mistake and went from thinking that to believing it. I was absolutely sure that the lab had mixed my tissue with someone else's sample. Even on April 19, 1975, the day of my mastectomy, I believed the diagnosis was a mistake. As they wheeled me into the operating room, I asked the doctor once again to check the pathology slides.

"I took out twenty-six lymph nodes, and they were all 'clean," the surgeon said after surgery, coming into my hospital room to tell me the news.

He was elated, but after he left I burst out crying. I was right: They had made a mistake after all. There was no cancer at all, and they had removed my breast for nothing. It took a while for me to accept the truth: There had been no mistake. Clean lymph nodes did not mean the absence of cancer, but that the cancer seemed not to have spread. Diagnosis: Stage I breast cancer. Circumscribed.

There are two ways to be a survivor in this world, two

modes that are quite different in their approaches to life. The first is best characterized by the Hebrew saying "If I am not there for me, who will be?" Fundamentally, this is a very insecure stance in the world, replete with bitterness and even hostility. This is a battle stance, an assumption that, with the worst yet to come, to let down the defenses even a little bit will let in a tide of unbearable misery and pain. This mode, employed to survive a crisis, uses up a substantial amount of physical and emotional energy.

The second mode is based on an assumption of abundance in the world: "God is behind me." This assumes support, so that when I'm challenged I'm just going to go for it. I don't have to survive on sheer willpower, because God has put wind in my sails. Surviving by sailing on God's power, having faith in the endless energy of the universe, creates physical and emotional energy.

But I didn't know about this second mode during those early years of cancer. I adopted the first, survivor mode, the stiff-upper-lip attitude that cancer is an unfortunate occurrence. The diagnosis of Stage I breast cancer marks what I call "Phase I" of my illness: I put my faith in medicine, was a "good" patient, and worked at recovery as though it were another goal to achieve, like earning a doctorate. With what I thought was admirable stoicism, I never talked about the cancer. I started swimming right away to regain the full use of my left arm, and I kept plugging away at my research. Chemotherapy was not given to Stage I breast cancer patients during those years, so Mike and I just figured the whole thing had come and gone.

Meanwhile, my career was proceeding very satisfactorily. I was finishing the last details of my Ph.D. in psychology, which I was awarded in 1978, and was interesting myself in the question of schizophrenia. I have always been interested in how people thought and felt, and came from Israel originally to study the psychology of interrelationships. My interest expanded to cognitive and perceptual problems and how the brain pro-

cesses information, and finally to understanding the schizo-
phrenic brain.

While involved with those questions, Mike and I were
preparing for marriage. Then, unexpectedly, in March 1978, a
spot on a rib showed up on a bone scan. We didn't know if
the spot was new or if it had been there quite a while.
Perhaps, we theorized hopefully, the spot hadn't shown up
on earlier scans because they had been done with older, less
refined equipment. But in the fall of 1979 a second spot
appeared on the scans; shortly after that, I was having back
pain, and my medical team diagnosed garden-variety breast
cancer, metastasized to the bone. That diagnosis of bone
metastases finally eradicated the last shred of doubt I might
have held onto, any remaining question I might have had
about the correctness of the initial diagnosis.

In the spring of 1980, I began my first round of chemotherapy, 10 cycles over 15 months. The idea was to just blast
those cells out of existence with an incredibly powerful treatment. This was not the standard medical therapy usually applied
in cases similar to mine. In fact, my doctor consulted other
specialists, who counseled not to do anything because, they
thought, I might be dead soon anyway. But my doctor believed
I could be cured, and I joined him in that belief.

The series was difficult, even brutal at times, but the effort
seemed worthwhile when, halfway through the treatments in
the spring of 1981, the bone scans showed no spots. I survived
the treatments because I believed they were working.

I believed then that I had made it, that, with the help of
science, I was cured. The pain was gone, the spots were gone,
and my confidence was back. Mike and I, along with the medical
team, celebrated the treatment as a great success.

Six months later the back pain returned and the spots
reappeared in the bone scans. That recurrence cracked, for a
second time, the illusion of being cured. This was a very crucial
point for me, in my illness and in my life. Suddenly I realized

that maybe medicine could do nothing for me. With this reappearance of the bone metastases, I entered a period of panic and depression that would bring about a major shift in attitude.

Until 1982, I had assumed that Western medicine would cure the illness if I followed my doctor's suggestions, kept up my interest in my career, and talked about my illness with no one outside a close circle of family and friends. Most of my research colleagues had no idea I had metastasized cancer. My sense then was that this silence was a good coping mechanism, since I didn't want to give cancer permission to change my life. I didn't join a support group, which I imagined as filled with people who weren't coping, who were sitting around feeling sorry for themselves. I wasn't going to be a complainer.

Outwardly, my career proceeded. I continued working at my research, writing papers about eye movement and schizophrenia, and preparing grant applications to maintain the financial support I needed for my research. I applied for and was granted the Research Scientist Development Award, an important five-year career development award given to a small number of promising young scientists, which allowed me to continue my research without constant worry over funding.

But at the same time, I knew I had cancer. I knew it was spreading and there was nothing I could do about it. When the medical treatments failed, I experienced a special kind of panic feeling, that control of my own destiny no longer lay in my own hands. I felt I was in a car with no driver, speeding faster and faster downhill, out of control.

Over the summer, that summer of panic, my initial stoic attitude in the face of cancer gave way to a new attitude. I was desperate to get rid of the helpless feeling. Until that summer, I thought it was my doctor's job to destroy the cancer and my job to research schizophrenia. I did not doubt that my doctor could do his job, and it did not occur to me to take part in the healing of my own body, other than to follow medical advice and keep the chemotherapy appointments.

But when the spots returned and I realized that the medical treatments had failed, I started looking for something I could do to help myself. Someone gave me the book *Recalled to Life*. Anthony J. Sattilaro, M.D., then president of Philadelphia's Methodist Hospital, claimed that a macrobiotic diet first relieved the pain of metastasized prostate cancer and then actually cured the cancer.

It seemed to me this guy Sattilaro had managed to grab the steering wheel and drive the car straight up the cliff, back onto the highway. As a scientist, I knew one case doesn't prove a thesis, but I intended to be the second case. I was impressed, but quickly became depressed. Macrobiotics would require me to give up the foods I loved most in the world: sweets, ice cream, sugar. Mike's favorite meal was corn chips, salsa, and beer.

Macrobiotics emphasized brown rice and seaweed. I spent one weekend being absolutely depressed, and then, Smadar-style, I gave away all my food, took cooking lessons, got books. How could I not reach out, I asked myself. How could I bear to lie on my deathbed and know that I was dying because I wouldn't give up ice cream?

Beginning the macrobiotic diet marks the end of the first phase of my illness and the beginning of the second. In Phase I, I was approaching the whole thing from an exclusively rational point of view. I saw cancer as an unfortunate mishap, something that happened to me. My strength came from not crashing under it, being a survivor in that negative, hostile way.

I characterize Phase II as guided by a "light-at-the-end-of-the-tunnel" mentality: A cure lay just around the corner, if only I could find where to turn in the maze. I shifted, psychologically, in that I began to ask what I had to do with the cancer. Why did I have this in my life? I understood, finally, that the cancer was more than an accident. But I still felt that my goal had to be to make the cancer go away, that I could find a way to cure myself, although medicine had failed to cure me. I felt I could only be fully happy when the cancer disappeared.

However, changing to a macrobiotic diet brought me, unexpectedly, to the threshold of another world: a world of energy and thus of God. I had thought of macrobiotic eating as allopathic medicine: Do this, and the cancer will be cured. I approached macrobiotic eating in the same way that I approached grant writing, relying on my achievement-oriented personality. But I learned through macrobiotics that there are truths other than the laws of scientific understanding.

I had never before thought of energy in a universal sense, over and above the mechanical interplay of specific forces described by Western physics. Macrobiotics is an Eastern philosophy that teaches that, for the body to be healthy, food types must be healthy and balanced. Too much yin energy in the food, or too much yang energy, can shock the body out of its essential balance.

Thinking about health and my own physical body in this new fashion opened the way for the first time for me to think about the universe and about my place in the universe. I learned that energy in the universe is also balanced between yin and yang, and that energy manifests itself on many levels aside from the physical, the most obvious level. And I learned that for energy to manifest itself on that most obvious level, it must already have manifested itself on less obvious emotional and spiritual planes.

And it is only a short step from believing in energy to believing in God. This was not someone saying, "Believe in God. It will make you feel better." This was a principle I could understand, apply to my daily life and use to connect myself to the universe: "expansion and contraction of energy." In Western culture, we think of God as an actual Being, a ruling king who sits in heaven and interacts with humans. God as Energy is a very different concept. I could finally see the connection between the energy of my physical body and the energy of the universe.

My vistas widened considerably. Previously I had considered science to be the truth. Now I know that science is a truth—an important, essential, and useful truth—but it is only one of many legitimate paths a person may choose to follow.

I followed macrobiotics strictly for more than a year—and in that time became a very healthy cancer patient—but my cancer continued to progress. I was at first quite upset that I couldn't make my cancer go away just by eating a strict macrobiotic diet. I was relying on my understanding of linear causality: This particular action will achieve that specific goal. Take this pill and that bacteria will disappear. Or eat these foods and that cancer will go away.

But causality is not that simple. We look at the world as though there is time: Monday comes before Tuesday. And as though there is simple linear causality: Kick a football and it goes into the goal. Those are only the frameworks of knowledge that we have devised to help us understand the world. There are so many other levels that we cannot see, of which we have no perception. There are other planes of perception outside of the very narrow limitations of the material plane. The point is, I learned I couldn't use macrobiotics as though it were medicine. Learning that lesson began a process of looking at all of life in a much more complex way.

While I was beginning to explore this new world, I continued my research and my career. By February 1985, I had finished my internship in neuropsychology at the Boston Veterans Administration Medical Center and was back working in the lab. With the career pressure, my diet and my energy level suffered, and I became ill enough that I had to stay in bed to regain strength. While I was in bed, I missed an opportunity to participate in authoring an important research paper on schizophrenia and genetics with two colleagues.

I reacted so strongly to the event—I felt I had a significant role in collecting the data for this paper and I fully expected to be included in its inception—that, for the first time, I had to look at my career goals and my own drive to achieve. How important was it to be an author on a paper about the genetics of schizo-phrenia? To drive myself to publish enough papers? Was I really happy in the lab, or was I conforming to an ideal of achievement?

What was obvious to me was that I was driving much harder than was good for me. The stress I was creating in my life was having a deleterious effect on my health. I cried and cried, agonizing. Finally I decided I was going to leave the lab. Technically I wasn't "leaving," that is "quitting." I was taking an unofficial leave of absence. But to me it felt like leaving, since I was entering a sort of limbo of unstructured living for the first time in my life. With that decision, I realized for the first time how much of me was tied up in external success, to the detriment of my internal self.

I took six months off to concentrate on my self-healing. I was eating strictly, meditating regularly. For the first time in my life, I left the straight-and-narrow goal-oriented path I had chosen and could just get up in the morning and read, sit alone with myself, go to the Cape, go and have a massage. I rested psychologically as well as physically, and my cancer retreated.

So then the question became, shouldn't I go back to work? Since I still didn't want to use the cancer as an "excuse," I agreed to go back to work three afternoons a week, and to work on my research at home the rest of the time.

This was agony, because I didn't feel connected to the work at the lab anymore. I had crossed some invisible boundary, entered another level of life. Soon after my return to the lab, October 1985, I had a diagnosis of metastases to the liver. I became extremely weak, sometimes barely able to move. After a trip to Israel to see my father in November, I became sicker.

It looked, for the first time, as though I might be dying. I was limping, losing weight, suffering from strange high fevers. My ribs kept breaking. I couldn't bend down to tie my shoes.

At that time I had a close friend, Susan, who was dying from inflammatory breast cancer. At Christmas, she rose from a coma long enough to return home from the hospital to be with her husband and two children. But in February, she returned to the hospital to die.

I went with her. I sat by her bed, held her hand, and listened as she talked about her feelings about dying. She knew I wasn't about to get terrified by anything she could tell me. And when she was in a coma, I talked to her. I know she listened.

While Susan was dying, her family asked me many questions. How to be with her while she was in the coma. What to say about all the morphine the hospital wanted to administer. How to deal with so many other medical and personal questions that come up around dying in a hospital. Everyone was as involved as possible, despite the hospital setting, and her death was an example of how beautiful the experience can be when everyone is communicating about it.

"You have the ability to look death in the face and walk through," my oncologist told me after my friend died.

He admired my behavior, but thought it strange. Like all doctors, Lee feels illness and death are bad things, things to cure, to make go away. But I felt I would be dying myself, soon, and I wanted to know what happens. I needed to see the physical vicissitudes of the dying process: What does the body look like? What physical processes occur? What happens when the liver goes? What happens in the hospital itself? What medications might be used? There are so many details, and I wanted to know as many of them as possible, to prepare myself for the shock.

For me, much of the fear of death, at a certain level, comes from not knowing, from being shot off my feet. One of my coping strategies from the beginning has been knowing what's going to happen when I go into the hospital. Moreover, I don't believe it's hard to face death. What's difficult is to be in the sorrow and sadness of people left behind. And I knew I had to stay with Susan. If you love someone, you can't quit at the last moment. I hope people won't do that to me.

After Susan's death, I realized I had important spiritual work I wanted to do. I had come light-years from the person I had been when first diagnosed at 28. But I realized there were elements of the spirit I had not yet begun to penetrate. Look at where I was that winter:

Reality I—medical: liver deteriorates, patient losing function.

Reality II—personal healing: When I returned to work, I relaxed my program, overdid activities, ate carelessly, stopped meditating regularly. You just can't take a few weeks off from such a healing program.

Reality III—emotional: Yielding to my own psychological pressure, I was working too hard, writing papers and working to achieve goals that were no longer essentially important to my inner life. I felt confused because few of my old friends and colleagues understood how greatly my sense of priorities had changed.

Reality IV—spiritual: I was in a sort of spiritual no-man's land, knowing that I needed to understand more about the life of the spirit, but not knowing how to go about that task.

If you ask why I got sick that winter, right before Susan's death, there are many ways to answer the question. The factors were scientific, holistic, emotional, spiritual. Basically, I was losing faith and losing focus.

I renewed my commitment to live when I set myself the goal of attaining a deeper spiritual understanding. I began planning for my fortieth birthday party in October 1986 and began another series of chemotherapy treatments. But after the first treatment I felt so drained of the will to live that I told my doctor I wouldn't take any more. I wanted some spunk left in me as I left the earth.

Sneaky Lee. He kept saying, "Just one more cycle." The horrible dead feeling after the first treatment came from all the dead cells leaving the body, he told me.

"You're just chock full of toxins," the doctor told me. "It

takes the luster out of you, but it means you're getting better. It will go away."

Just one more, he said. And I took another, and another. The second treatment was better and the third was even better, just like he promised. The tumor melted away. When we started, my CEA (a diagnostic test believed to measure the amount of tumor in the body) was at 250; when we completed the series it had dropped to 40.

In December 1986, little more than a year after the metastatic liver diagnosis, I had another scan. The spots on my bones were so numerous that they lit up the scan like a Christmas tree. Despite those tests, I spent the next several months studying intensely, in order to pass my clinical counseling exam so that I could begin to work with cancer patients and other clients.

In April of 1987, I passed the exam and met the spiritual guide who would begin preparing me for the trip to Brazil. During this year another shift in my understanding began, a shift so subtle and nonverbal that even now I find it difficult to understand and explain. But I am sure of one thing: My growing faith provided the energy to overcome the liver metastases.

That spring and summer I was very, very ill and spent a considerable amount of time in bed. In June and July I visited a psychic healer four times: He put his hands on my head. The CEA numbers didn't go down, but the fevers stopped and I felt stronger.

"Nothing is stronger than God's energy," he told me in August 1987 when I asked about beginning another chemotherapy series. "When you go back to Boston, when you start the new chemotherapy, it's going to work very well, because God's energy is there."

It was like someone flipped the switch. I had a tiny weekly allotment of adriamycin, beginning in August 1987, and somehow I got a new lease on life. I had enough energy to spend the next year establishing a cancer counseling center with two colleagues, to travel to Brazil seeking a deeper spiritual understanding, and to learn to ride a horse.

Again we have the question of realities. The medical reality is: The adriamycin worked. My doctor's reality is: A certain class of patients, those who take charge, do well. He sees the issue as one of psychological control, and doesn't think it matters what I do, as long as I have an emotional sense of control.

My reality is this: My renewed commitment for further spiritual growth and self-healing made the adriamycin work. I had more things to learn on this earth, and, spiritually, I was not ready to die.

Although I have not been "cured" of cancer, I have come to understand that I have been seeking—and have begun achieving—a "healing." "Healing" means to be made whole again, and I have experienced a growing understanding of what that means. By no means is my understanding complete. For me, healing is not an end state, but a process that has to do with continuously coming to express and manifest and be who I truly am in my most natural, whole, divine self.

Phase III of my illness, acceptance that I could live the remaining days of my life with cancer in my body, began a bit after the liver diagnosis, with the beginning of the chemo series, in January 1988. I accepted the fact that I might die soon, but I also made a commitment to heal and to try to live as full a life as I could with the cancer in my body. I came to terms with the fact that I might have to live with the cancer for a long, long time, and couldn't continue to put my life on hold until it was gone. I decided that although I might never be free of cancer, I would live a very full life.

I don't know how to characterize the fourth phase, which started only last winter when I came back from Brazil. It looked like I was running out of medical options, and I started to think about surrendering. The experience in the spiritual community in Brazil helped me understand the difference between giving in, which I have never done, and surrendering, which I realized I needed to explore. You see, as long as I was struggling with death to hold it off, to hold it at bay, I was feeding the fear and feeding the death. In Brazil I learned that I needed to let divine help in, and open up to divinity's possibilities.

EPILOGUE

Smadar died on January 19, 1989.

In 1987, Smadar founded the Wellspring Center for Life Enhancement, a cancer-counseling center in Watertown, Massachusetts, with several colleagues.

Smadar asked her oncologist at the Dana Farber Cancer Institute to participate in this book, but he refused to do so. One co-founder, who worked with Smadar for many years as both physician-counselor and colleague, did speak about Smadar's case at her request.

"Smadar's case is unusual from two perspectives, the physical and the psychospiritual," he said, just before her death. "Most people with bone metastases from breast cancer don't live more than 5 years from the onset of the illness. Here we are, 14 years later. Those with liver metastases generally don't live more than 6 to 12 months from the onset of metastases. Here she is, 3 years later. Smadar is, in all these areas, an exception, at the end of the bell curve of survival.

"But this is certainly not the most significant aspect of her healing. Healing has more to do with the quality of life than it has to do with longevity of the body. If we equate success with the survival of the body, then we're all failures. We all die.

"Smadar's story is the story of a young Israeli woman,

very intelligent and a high-need achiever, who gets married and discovers at the same time that she has cancer, and who uses the course of her illness as a path of spiritual awakening and self-healing. In the process, she becomes a teacher of the principles of holistic healing.

"Her option for a bone marrow transplant was eliminated, and chemotherapy had nothing more to offer. Yet she continued to work and to live her life, counseling other cancer patients and teaching us all. Here is someone who has made a heroic attempt to heal her body, and in the process has healed her mind."

Sylvia Johnson

INTRODUCTION

In March 1980, Sylvia Johnson lay in a hospital bed in Los Angeles, in intense pain from a massive tumor that extended from her neck, under her arm, into her torso. The tumor, the fourth major recurrence of breast cancer in less than a year, was so large surgeons couldn't operate to remove it. Neither had the tumor responded to radiation or chemotherapy treatments.

The hospital's social worker had already begun talking with Sylvia's two daughters about their mother dying. Sylvia's husband, after several discouraging discussions with her doctor, had little hope.

Sylvia herself started to look at dying as an alternative to the overwhelming pain. She felt herself losing her will to live.

Sylvia's Story

Like life itself, the will to live is a subtle thing. For many years before my cancer diagnosis, I unconsciously lacked that will, living in a most self-destructive way. But by the time my cancer appeared, I had begun to acknowledge my self-hatred and change my life-style. My husband and I had both stopped drinking and had dedicated our lives to being of service and to a Higher Power. We were at peace for the first time in many years, and our two daughters were so happy for us.

And then the cancer came. In March 1979, I was 48 years old, a wife for 28 years and a founder and teacher at the Plymouth School for preschoolers. I had been a public school teacher back in New England, where Major, my husband, and I both came from. But in Los Angeles, public school positions were rare.

With several others, I founded the Plymouth School, to teach children self-esteem and social adjustment. The school was a success—it still is—but I could never earn as much money as I would have in the public schools. To make up the deficit, I ran all around the city at night teaching speed reading. My daughters, my husband, and my home also required time and attention. As Superwoman, I tried to do it all.

I was exhausted from overwork, frustration, misdirected anger, and a sort of general disappointment with life. Those feelings manifested themselves in a growing problem with alcohol, which only made everything 10 times worse. We had finally faced that problem—Major a bit sooner than I—and we both have been sober ever since. One day I felt a lump in my right breast. For months, I had been thinking about having a checkup, but I didn't even have a doctor. Then I read a magazine article about self-examination and, following instructions, I felt the breast and found the lump.

At school I told another teacher, who insisted I do something about it. On the way home from school, I stopped at a phone booth and started dropping in dimes, calling around to find someone to see. I wasn't even sure what kind of doctor I should contact.

After giving me a mammogram, a radiologist said the lump could be malignant and suggested a biopsy. After the biopsy, the surgeon woke me in the recovery room to tell me the lump was malignant. Just like that, in that instant, my whole life changed forever.

I flew apart. I can't say I was brave or stoic at all. I screamed and hollered and cried, and the nurse tried to comfort me. I took three days to get used to the idea of losing a body part and to the idea that I had a life-threatening illness. Then I was back in the hospital for the surgery. There wasn't too much question about having the breast removed. In those days, the possibilities of treatment were so narrow. Mastectomies were about it.

Before the mastectomy, I went off by myself to say good-bye to my breast. It was my favorite one, and the disease wasn't her fault. I felt so sad. The surgeon removed 15 lymph nodes along with the breast, and found disease in four of them.

Radiation and chemotherapy, administered by an oncologist who was a real authority-figure, followed the surgery. I cried a lot about having cancer, but I believed the doctors when they said I had a good chance, at my age, for a total cure. The oncologist insisted on immediate compliance with his protocol, and I followed his orders.

But the cancer came back in December. A site in the chest wall right under the mastectomy scar had become cancerous. Another surgery was required. I was terribly frightened this time.

"I'm so worried," I told the surgeon.

"I know lots of women with recurrences who have done quite well," he reassured me.

Then, in February, there were more lumps, lumps in the lymph nodes on the right side. This time I felt it would never stop, that the cancer was a team of wild horses dragging me off and that I couldn't help myself anymore. Back in the hospital the third time, for a third surgical operation, the feeling of helplessness was just awful. I am a fighter, with plenty of spirit and anger. But the helplessness I felt from this onslaught seemed to take much of the fight out of me. Who is strong enough to fight trampling horses?

In March, I got up one morning and felt a lump the size of a golf ball on the left side of my neck.

"Can this be?" I asked myself. "Can this really be happening again?"

I was very, very depressed. I went off to school and asked another teacher if she felt anything.

"I think you'd better have it checked out," she said, with tears in her eyes, looking so frightened.

"I just don't want to know anymore," I thought to myself.

I wanted very much to believe it was just scar tissue, so for a short while I put off seeing a doctor. But, depressed and discouraged as I was, something made me take action. Examining the lump, my oncologist suspected the tumor extended all the way down my side. A biopsy showed malignancy, but the tumor was inoperable—too much body tissue was involved this time.

During those days and nights I lay on the couch in our apartment, sometimes facing the wall, sometimes facing the room, always trying to find a way to escape the pain. Pain filled my whole body, consumed my whole conscious life. I could find no way to be comfortable or at ease in any way.

"Will you please let me put you in the hospital?" my oncologist begged. "You are in so much pain that your body can't begin to heal. At least go into the hospital so I can prescribe methadone and ease your pain."

Despite my agony, I refused for a long time. When I went into the hospital this time, I knew I wouldn't come out.

"Cancer is a team of horses running away with me," I repeated to myself. "There's no way back this time."

Finally, I gave in.

"I can't do this myself. I can't bear this any longer," I told Major.

I left my apartment, perhaps for the last time, and went into the hospital. No one said I was dying at that time, but everyone was thinking it. Our two girls were at college, and everyone was very frightened. They came home from school to be with me.

"If we can't find something that works, you'll probably only have a few months to live," the doctor said.

When he said it, I didn't really hear it. I kept asking Major over and over again if that was really what the doctor said.

The plan was to give me methadone and thorazine first, to ease the pain and help relax my body, and then to give me a super dose of chemotherapy, following an experimental protocol. This was a kind of last-ditch effort, a massive combination of superdrugs designed to flood my body and wash out all the cancer cells.

But first, I had to take the methadone. I had spent a long time teaching myself not to cover up psychological pain by resorting to alcohol. The methadone felt like a real defeat to me, since I felt I should also be able to handle physical pain without resorting to a drug. Taking the drug, I felt, was giving in to weakness and admitting that I might be dying.

The first night I was in the hospital, the night before I was to take my first methadone dose, a male nurse came in. For some reason I started talking to him even though I didn't know him.

"The doctor wants me to take methadone," I said. "But I've just gotten sober. I'm afraid this will start everything up all over again."

"I'm a recovered addict, and I can understand what your fears are," he answered, taking my hand and speaking softly and gently. "You can't heal with all this pain. You need first to take the methadone and get better. We'll turn this over to a Higher Power. This is not yours to decide. It will be what it will be."

His words put me at ease. I believed him, and realized that the matter was no longer under my control. I don't believe this man's presence in my room, and his calm faith, were accidental or coincidental. I believe he was with me that night by God's grace, to help me make a difficult decision.

Although I agreed to take the methadone, I was, in my heart, questioning the value of life itself. During those first pain-filled days in the hospital, when I had given up trying to stay in my own home and when I had consented to take the drug, I was no longer sure I wanted to live.

"How can life be worth living, with so much pain and so many problems?" I asked myself. "Can I continue to go through this, with no end in sight? Even if this lump goes away, another will come soon after to take its place."

The seemingly endless succession of lumps, surgery, radiation, chemotherapy, and mind-dulling drugs was all I could see in life. Some part of me then was walking a precipice, considering an ultimate decision. I could step over the edge, into the abyss, and not be troubled anymore. During that time, I came to understand that death is not so much to be feared, when the time comes.

The doctors, my children, and my husband were waiting to see how I would respond to treatment. I know that I was hovering myself, looking into the abyss and making some sort of decision, trying to gather strength for one more try. But the strength just wasn't there.

One night I woke with a start. I felt a big ball of fire burning in my chest. The burning was not painful, but it was strong and dominating and unavoidable. It was a kind of glowing energy which seemed to want to subsume all of my body. My heart beat unbelievably fast. I was very frightened.

"I'm dying now," I thought. "This is it. The choice is made."

Then I was so surprised. Suddenly I understood: The opposite was true. The message was absolute and a choice had been made, I was right about that. But I was wrong about the choice itself.

I was absolutely going to live. The flash of energy lasted several minutes. For me, that energy was a message from my Higher Power. There was no God in flowing robes, no burning bush or visible sign. There was just a simple but powerful feeling of love and energy.

I lay awake the rest of the night, thinking about what this meant. I began to feel that I could survive. Whether to live or die was no longer a question. The question remaining to me was: How would I live the life given to me?

The will to live had a lot to do with my recovery. One of my doctors scoffs when I say that, but I know it's true. Having the will to live doesn't necessarily mean I would recover. But without that will, recovery is impossible.

From that night on, I feel that I started improving medically. I don't know what the medical facts are; I can't speak in medical terms. I can only say what I myself felt.

The experience was a signal: Get going on survival. Begin immediately.

I spent six weeks in the hospital that time, drugged from the methadone and washed out from the chemotherapy. That hospital room was so dreary, but we worked hard to brighten it up. Major brought in all the stuffed animals he could find, and kept buying more and more. Our study at home is filled with them now. My roommate came from a large Korean family that grew orchids. Her orchids and my animals filled the window sills and the corners, and we put bright pictures on the walls. Major put up my favorite picture of the ocean at sunset.

Before cancer, I liked hospitals. I had had my babies in hospitals and had fun both times. But by now I had come to loathe the corridors and the smells and the rules and regulations. I developed a fixation on the fire escape, dreaming about climbing out the window and down the escape to the street.

"The nurse will never know," I told myself. "She's too far away at the other end of the hall to catch me."

Of course, I was too weak to do anything. In those first weeks Major came in the morning before work, to feed me and to read to me from our spiritual books. Two incredibly faithful friends came every day in the middle of the day. One woman fed me lunch each day, since I was too weak to feed myself. Another woman came each day at noon, on her lunch hour. We didn't talk, but through the fog I could feel her each day pick up my hand and stand there quietly, thinking about me.

The massive tumor melted away. And I regained my strength. At night I'd get really terrified. I'd go to the door of the room, wanting to walk up and down the hall, just to get out of my prison. But the night nurse wouldn't let me out into the hall, so I'd stand at the window and look down at the Café Santa Monica across the street.

"If I ever get out of here," I thought, "I'll go over there and have a cup of coffee."

My doctor finally allowed me to go home. He never said anything definitive about the cancer, that I was cured or cancer free.

"Go home and give it a try" was his pronouncement. But I know he was surprised, along with everyone else.

That was the last tumor I had. In nine years, the cancer has not reappeared.

Yet I know that cancer cells could still be inside my body and that developing another tumor is always possible. And so I live my life differently now. I concentrate on maintaining a healthy immune system, one that is able to fight the microscopic cells before they get out of control and overwhelm my body again. The lesson of that night is that I have been given special, extra time on this earth, and that I must guard that time carefully.

As soon as I became strong enough, I attended meetings

and group sessions at the Center for the Healing Arts. The center, which no longer exists, taught that physical health depends on psychological health, and that we can't have one without the other.

Since childhood, I had experienced irrational fits of rage, when I would yell and scream and throw things against the wall. When I wasn't angry, I was terrified, terrified something would happen to my children or to my husband. If Major was back an hour or two late from a trip, he would come home to find me either convinced he had died in an auto accident or convinced he had left me for another woman.

At the center, we discovered for the first time why I felt this way. When I was seven years old, my father died. I had never accepted his death, and never stopped being angry, as only a child can be, about being abandoned.

To say that this unconscious anger directly caused the cancer is, admittedly, a giant step. But to say that the anger caused much of the misery and terror and irrational rage is, I think, quite believable. And to say that those feelings caused behaviors that hurt me physically as well as emotionally is also, I think, quite believable.

At the very least, the anger helped cause the drinking, since I was clearly trying to dull these frightening, uncontrollable feelings. And the drinking, of course, created all kinds of physical as well as emotional problems.

I believe that psychological health directly affects physical health. As an adult, I felt silly being angry with my father for dying. He couldn't help it; I'm sure the heart attack wasn't his idea. Still, I had to work through my childish anger and forgive him.

In the process, I learned about working through anger with others, a skill that has been essential in maintaining my health. It's extremely stressful, and therefore unhealthy, to stuff feelings away until they come out in a rage. And for cancer patients, stuffing feelings is a very dangerous process.

But when I admitted that the child in me was still angry, the anger went away. And with its dissolution, my own rages and terrors largely disappeared. I still get angry, but in a normal and healthy way. I don't throw things at the wall, and I don't try to hurt myself by drinking alcohol or smoking cigarettes or eating too much.

And I don't try to be Superwoman anymore. I am satisfied to be me. I teach half-days at the school now, and I don't teach at night at all. The family has adjusted to the smaller income, and my life is in better balance. I do some work with our spiritual group and help others who are trying to stop drinking. I also work with cancer patients, helping them believe, through my own example, that even the worst cases of cancer can have unpredictable outcomes.

I don't know what caused that last tumor to disappear. You do everything you can, fight as hard as you can, with whatever is available. And then you accept the outcome, whatever it is. Perhaps there is some ultimate plan, but it's a plan that we are not meant to understand. I have my own ideas about that particular night, when I felt myself hovering at the abyss, but I can't prove them. My doctor, I'm sure, has his own ideas about what saved my life. Those ideas are also unprovable.

But I am certain of one thing. My own behavior and my own attitudes have made the quality of my life a thousand percent better. And I think they've helped to keep my cancer from recurring. At any rate, I have been at the abyss, and I've decided life is worth living.

I volunteer weekly at the Wellness Community, a non-profit cancer support agency, telling newly diagnosed patients my story.

"If you're well, why do you dwell on it? Why do you keep digging all this stuff up again?" some people ask.

"It keeps me well to remember where I came from," is my answer.

It's a matter of gratitude, and a good way to keep the lessons I've learned in the forefront of my life. Even after eight years now, there's no way to know whether I'll wake up again one morning with a tumor. So I take one day at a time. I don't have any expectations for the future, but appreciate what comes my way.

Several years ago, my daughter Caroline married.

"I never thought you'd be alive to see this wedding," my brother told me with tears in his eyes.

This past year, on November 30, 1988, to be exact, Caroline gave birth to our first grandchild. To have your own child give birth to a child is an experience that is truly miraculous. Now I am a grandmother.

And this summer, Major, an ordained Baptist minister, will officiate at our second daughter's wedding. Perhaps we will have another grandchild in the next few years.

There are things going on here that I know nothing about. I think God makes these decisions, and, for now, this is how I fit into things. This is probably a pretty simplistic view, but this is how I see it.

We have choices about how to live. But we don't have the ultimate choice. That's not how it's supposed to be.

EPILOGUE

Sylvia's oncologist, David Plotkin of Los Angeles, said he was very surprised that Sylvia's tumor responded to the experimental chemotherapy he prescribed. Other patients using that therapy, Plotkin said, did not respond nearly as well.

"Sylvia's disease was bad. It was not widespread, but largely confined to the mastectomy side. However, it had proved resistant to all treatments, until this last one I gave her.

"Her Karnofsky Performance Status [a measure of physical ability] was about 60 to 70 percent.* She was not cadaverous. She was up and about and ambulating. Nevertheless, she did have a mass of biopsy-proven tumor tissue that had proven resistant to standard therapy and radiation therapy. I gave her this experimental stuff I was using at the time and she responded brilliantly.

"More importantly, she has continued in remission. It's this staying respondent that's really one for the books. She was certainly not a cadaver, but she was Stage IV. When people have that kind of extensive disease they have microscopic disease elsewhere. It can't be proven, obviously, since it can't be seen. But generally, within several months, evidence of widespread disseminated disease becomes evident.

"This lady had incredible biological luck. If a woman has breast cancer, far better that she should have great luck biologically than smart doctors. I've been an oncologist for 30 years, and I've seen a lot of things happen. I'm not struck by the fact that one's attitude has a lot to do with this. I have seen misanthropes do well, and those filled with tremendous love and family support go down the tubes.

"Sylvia was luckier than hell. The basis for people thinking attitude has something to do with it is all part of a myth of control. Everyone wants to control their lives, and it's just a lot of BS. If you want to control your life with respect to health, avoid smoking or being overweight or riding on a motorcycle without a helmet. But the big issues, what's going to happen ultimately, all that is controlled by stuff like DNA.

---

* The Karnofsky scale measures a set of performance criteria to ascertain the seriousness of a person's physical illness: 100 is normal; 10 is moribund, unable to care for self.

"*The fact that she responded so incredibly to it was amazing. It was outhouse luck. It wasn't because of her attitude or because I'm such a good doctor. It was just outhouse luck.*"

Epilogue

Just as I was finishing this book, a guest came to stay at our house. We didn't know him well, and he laid it right on the line the moment he walked in the door.

"Let's just get this out, right from the beginning: I have cancer," he said, not knowing about this book.

"What kind of cancer do you have?" I asked.

"Here," he said, pointing to his lungs.

"And here," he added, pointing to his head. "A double whammy. You can't get much worse than that."

He told me what had become by then a familiar litany: a diagnosis followed by admonishments to change diet and lifestyle followed by dire statistics and a warning to get his affairs in order.

"But I'm going to be different," he said. "I'm going to beat those statistics."

We talked about his strategy. He followed the doctor's recommendations for chemotherapy and radiation. He adopted a diet-oriented therapy based on the ideas of a New York doctor. He attended a cancer support organization. He meditated and used visualization each day. He also said he had faith that things would work out.

And he had a reason to live. Our friend and his wife had brought their 6-year-old granddaughter to Plymouth to celebrate the Fourth of July. They figured they'd do Plimoth Plantation and the *Mayflower*, get in a round of miniature golf, and top the day off with Fourth of July fireworks in America's Hometown.

While we were talking in the kitchen, the 6-year-old floated in and sat on her grandfather's lap. The child reached up and put her arms around the man's neck. Graced with his granddaughter's smile, the grandfather glowed.

"What you do is, you try everything," he said, as she ran outdoors. "You do what you can. And you remember to love."

This book is meant for all those who want to continue to love and to live, despite life's difficulties.

For more information, contact:

Wendy Williams
Box 14
Mashpee, MA 02649